Acknowledgements

The *Introductory Guide – NHS Finance* is developed under the direction of the HFMA's Financial Management and Research Committee and with the help of a wide range of practitioners, all of whom give their time and expertise free of charge. The HFMA is extremely grateful to everyone who has been involved in the Guide's production. The main contributors to this edition are:

Keith Wood (Chair of the committee)

Les Allen
Pen Andersen
Sarah Bence
Phil Bradley
Steve Brown
Mark Collis
Bernard Crotty
Michael Davies
Nigel Davies
Richard Edwards
Steve Elliot
Catherine Eyre
Janice Fawell
Nigel Foster
Nick Gerrard
Kavita Gnanaolivu
Anna Green
Paul Holland
Tom Jackson
Emma Knowles

Kate Mathers
Patrick McDermott
Richard Mellor
Glen Palethorpe
Debbie Paterson
Tracey Paton
Janet Perry
Sheenagh Powell
Antony Rodden
Pippa Ross-Smith
David Savage
Richard Sharp
Simon Sheppard
Bryn Shorney
Pat Shroff
Karl Simkins
Lindsay Stead
Helen Strain
Mike Townsend
Robert White

The editor is Anna Green.

Chapter 1: Introduction and Purpose

About the Guide

For more than twenty years, the *Introductory Guide to NHS Finance* has sought to provide an easy to read, accessible Guide to the workings and language of NHS finance for the benefit of practitioners and observers. The Guide is produced by The Healthcare Financial Management Association (HFMA), a charity established 60 years ago to support those working within the NHS finance function. By improving financial literacy both within and outside NHS finance, the HFMA hopes it can inform and improve the debate on healthcare finance issues.

The Guide has been developed to provide a self-contained source of advice and guidance for readers from an array of backgrounds. There are many aspects of NHS finance that are unique to the service, and a language laden with jargon, abbreviations and acronyms has developed that can appear impenetrable to many outsiders or newcomers. Indeed, as the terminology develops with each set of reforms, even the most experienced NHS finance professionals can find themselves in unfamiliar territory!

The Guide aims to provide advice to all levels of finance staff from finance directors (who often use it as an aide memoir to more recent changes) to governors and lay members; non-executive and executive directors (who may not be finance specialists but still have shared corporate responsibility for understanding and managing the financial position); clinicians; budget holders; service managers; accounts assistants and those who need an understanding of NHS finance for academic study purposes.

Over the years the Guide has grown in size as it tries to provide an overview of both the current finance regime along with a sense of how the approach has developed over the years. Nevertheless, it remains (as its title suggests) an introductory guide that gives a reasonably straightforward but comprehensive description of NHS structures and processes.

The last version of the Guide was produced in 2011 as the Coalition Government was preparing to implement a programme of proposals first set out in its June 2010 white paper *Equity and Excellence: Liberating the NHS* and passed into legislation by *The Health and Social Care Act 2012*. This has resulted in changes to the structure and approach of the NHS that are more dramatic than any other reforms since the NHS was established in 1948.

Approach and Format

This version of the *Introductory Guide* follows the approach readers will be familiar with – namely that each chapter treats its topic in a largely self-contained way. Cross-references are included where they are helpful and sources of further advice and technical guidance are listed at the end of each chapter. For the later chapters, there are also lists of 'key learning points'.

The bulk of the Guide concentrates on the financial arrangements for the NHS in England. There are also chapters highlighting key differences in Northern Ireland, Scotland and Wales – these differences are now even more marked as the 2012 Act applies only to England.

The Guide ends with a glossary of terms and abbreviations.

HFMA E-learning and the Introductory Certificate to NHS Finance

In addition to the *Introductory Guide*, the HFMA produces a series of e-learning courses that allow individuals to address their NHS finance training needs in a tailored way. The e-learning modules are aimed primarily at non-finance professionals including governors, lay members, non-executive directors, clinical staff, general practice staff and finance staff that are new to the NHS. They can also be used as 'refreshers' for existing staff.

Although modules can be studied individually, there is an *Introductory Certificate* that involves learners selecting five modules from an ever expanding list of topics. These cover both the structure of the NHS (for example, NHS finance, primary care finance and the foundation trust financial regime) and processes (for example, commissioning, budgeting and costing). Each training session takes between two and three hours to complete and includes an assessment test. On successful completion of the fifth module, an *Introductory Certificate to NHS Finance* is awarded – this is fast becoming an industry standard; a means of assessing an individual's basic competence in NHS finance. Further details are available from the HFMA website at www.hfma.org.uk

References and Further Reading

Equity and Excellence: Liberating the NHS, Department of Health, 2010: https://www.gov.uk/government/publications/liberating-the-nhs-white-paper

The Health and Social Care Act 2012: www.legislation.gov.uk/ukpga/2012/7/contents/enacted

Chapter 2: NHS Finance Background and Context – how we got to where we are today

Overview

This chapter looks back over recent years to chart the development of the NHS so that we can see how we have reached where we are in 2013. First we need to look at how and when the NHS began.

The Introduction of the NHS

The NHS was established by the *NHS Act 1946*. This Act specified that, it was 'the duty of the Minister… to promote the establishment in England and Wales of a comprehensive Health Service designed to secure the improvement of the physical and mental health of the people of England and Wales and the prevention, diagnosis and treatment of illness'. The services provided to meet these aims were to be free of charge, based on clinical need, not the ability to pay.

The NHS was launched and the first patients treated on 5 July 1948.

Underpinning Principles of the NHS

Although there have been many structural and policy developments since 1948, the underlying principles have not changed. These are that NHS services are:

* available to everyone
* free at the point of need (or use)
* based on clinical need, not the ability to pay.

All three main political parties remain committed to these core principles.

Other enduring characteristics of the NHS are that:

* it is funded through taxation
* it manages within overall resource limits determined by the Government each year
* finite resources have to be matched with infinite demand for health services with tough choices over priorities needed as a result
* there is an expectation that 'efficiency savings' can be made, often as a result of structural or technical developments
* there is intense political, public and media interest in, and scrutiny of, the NHS.

The NHS is also Europe's largest employer with over 1.5 million employees. However, although it is usually referred to as if it were a single organisation, it actually comprises a wide range of different bodies with specific responsibilities – we will be looking at many of these later on in the Guide.

Key Policy Developments that have Shaped the NHS since the 1980s

The internal market, 1980s

In the late 1980s it was decided that the NHS should be reconfigured along purchaser and provider lines. This required the NHS to operate a 'quasi-market', known as the internal market. The key feature of this approach was the separation of the provision of hospital and community services from the commissioning or purchasing function – the so-called 'purchaser/ provider split'. Hospitals were encouraged to apply for self-governing trust status, creating organisations quite separate from the health authorities from which they were devolved. To achieve trust status, and formally separate from the health authorities, provider organisations had to follow an application process that assessed viability and robustness.

There was also an optional scheme to give general practitioners (GPs) the ability to hold budgets for the purchase of hospital services for their patients (known as GP fund holding). At the same time, trusts were encouraged to invest in and develop services and to compete with each other to win patient service contracts with purchasers.

There were a number of criticisms associated with the internal market. In particular, it was argued that it led to fragmentation and a lottery in service provision, with competition proving a weak lever for improvement. It also led to overall increases in administration costs as 'losing' organisations had to be sustained to ensure that services could be maintained.

In 1997, the change of Government resulted in plans to dismantle the internal market.

The New NHS – Modern, Dependable, 1997

In 1997, the White Paper *The New NHS – Modern, Dependable* set out a programme for reform of the NHS. These proposals became law with the *1999 Health Act* (since superseded by the *NHS Act 2006*) and the focus shifted away from competition to a collaborative model, where NHS organisations worked together and with local authorities to re-focus healthcare on the patient. By removing the competitive nature of the internal market, the changes in policy sought to ensure the seamless delivery of services.

Key changes were an end to GP fund holding and the introduction of new organisations for primary care. Primary care organisations (either 'groups' or 'trusts') were formed from groups of local GP practices, or 'natural communities'. Boundaries were encouraged to coincide where possible with local authority borders to simplify the integration of health and social care. In their initial stages these groups were sub-committees of health authorities, used to inform the commissioning process. As they found their feet, they were able to apply for trust status, creating bodies independent from the health authority and managing increasingly significant portions of former health authority budgets.

The *1999 Health Act* also established the Commission for Health Improvement (to be succeeded by the Commission for Healthcare Audit and Inspection, then by the Healthcare Commission and now the Care Quality Commission) and the National Institute for Health and Clinical Excellence or NICE – now renamed the National Institute for Care and Excellence.

There was also a renewed emphasis on cutting management costs – a challenging objective given the increase in the number of NHS organisations, and greater involvement of management at a local level. The 'shared services initiative' was, at least to an extent, an attempt to mitigate the pressure on management costs by reducing the cost of providing support services (particularly 'back office' functions). National shared service centre pilots were established and there are now a number of shared business services centres around the country, run as a joint venture between the Department of Health and Steria.

The purchaser/provider split created by the internal market was retained. Initially health authorities remained and continued to purchase healthcare using 'service and financial framework agreements'. These health authorities were then abolished but the division between commissioning and provision continued with primary care trusts (PCTs) taking over responsibility for commissioning hospital services. At their inception, many PCTs also had a provider role in relation to community services.

The 1997 White Paper also heralded a move towards longer planning time frames, promising the replacement of annual contract negotiations with three-year resource announcements. This was delivered at a Department of Health level, with the budget announcement including levels of funding for the next three years. Three-year allocations to PCTs were introduced from 2003/04 to help improve the service planning process and most organisations committed to three-year local delivery plans – although the level of detail incorporated in years two and three was limited.

The NHS was encouraged to form partnerships with both private and public sector partners, including local authority social services. The *1999 Health Act* also broadened the scope for pooling of health and social services budgets. Partnership working with the private sector was formalised in a 'concordat' agreement, which highlighted scope for joint working in elective, critical and intermediate care. New independently run diagnosis and treatment centres or 'independent sector treatment centres' (ISTCs) were established so extending the role of the private sector in the NHS.

The NHS Plan: a Plan for Investment, a Plan for Reform, 2000

In July 2000 the *NHS Plan* was presented to Parliament. The plan consisted of a vision of the NHS first outlined in the 1997 White Paper – modernised, structurally reformed, efficient and properly funded. Much of the document was dedicated to identifying new targets and milestones on wide ranging issues (from waiting lists to implementation of electronic patient records) and measures that needed to be taken to facilitate the achievement of those targets.

The Health Act 2002

In April 2002 a further tranche of changes came into effect. At the end of March 2002, the 95 health authorities in England were abolished and replaced by 28 strategic health authorities (SHAs). At the same time the eight regional offices were replaced by four directorates of health and social care which were themselves dissolved in 2003. The changes, first outlined in April 2001 in the policy paper *Shifting the Balance of Power*, were designed to transfer management resource and control closer to the locality, and hence to the patient.

The establishment of PCTs was also completed in 2002 – a key change here was the fact that PCTs were allowed to expand primary care services beyond those traditionally provided by GPs. This prompted a growth in 'GPs with special interests' and in services provided in the community by PCTs where previously they had been delivered in an acute hospital setting.

Many of the monitoring and planning processes were devolved from the old regional offices to the new SHAs, while commissioning functions were transferred to PCTs.

The structure that was introduced in 2002 for the NHS in England is shown below. This included foundation trusts that came into being following the *Health and Social Care (Community Standards) Act 2003* (see later in this chapter) and lasted until March 2013.

NHS Structure 2002 to 2013

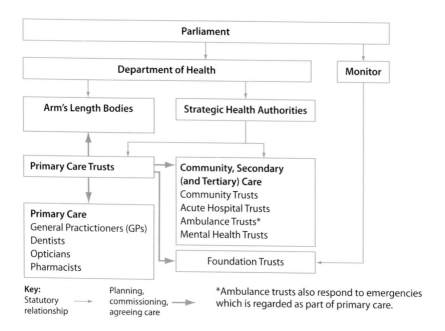

Comprehensive spending reviews and budgets

In terms of overall funding levels, the Labour Government made a commitment in 1997 to increasing NHS funding to a level that would bring the UK's health spending in line with the average for the rest of Europe. The first step toward this target was taken in the 2000 budget, with a further significant increase in 2001. However, it was the 2002 budget that gave the first indication of the substantial and long-term increases required if that promise was to be delivered. Funding for these increases was achieved by the introduction of employer and employee national insurance surcharges at a rate of 1%, and from the release of funds from other sources, enabled by the Government's comprehensive spending review (CSR). The CSR process is designed to assess critically the spending of government departments in the light of changing priorities.

Successive budgets maintained the commitment to longer-term budgeting. However, the 2007 CSR process led to more modest increases for the three year period from 2008/09 compared with the preceding period, averaging 3.9% growth in real terms, compared with 7.5% for the previous CSR period.

The impact of the economic downturn following the banking crisis in 2008 led to warnings about the future funding of the NHS. The *Pre-Budget Report 2009*, the 2010/11 *Operating Framework* and the *Budget 2010 – Securing the Recovery* began to highlight the extent of the challenge.

In preparation for tighter times ahead, efficiency savings targets steadily moved upwards. To help achieve these targets and in line with a renewed emphasis on quality, the Department of Health expected NHS organisations to meet the 'quality, innovation, productivity and prevention (QIPP) challenge'. In practice, this meant organisations had to follow 'lean management principles' of avoiding duplication, preventing errors that then need to be corrected, and stopping ineffective practices. Inevitably this involved a focus on reducing back office functions and (from a finance perspective) re-ignited the debate about the relative advantages and disadvantages of shared services.

The spending review that took place in October 2010 reflected the need to reduce significantly the public sector borrowing requirement. However, the health budget was protected with the result that revenue spending in England is due to rise to £109.8bn by 2014/15 (see chapter 10 for details).

Payment by results

A key element of the Labour Government's modernisation plans involved reforming the financial framework and the way funding flowed around the NHS. The proposal for bringing about this change was set out in 2002 in *Delivering the NHS Improvement Plan* and introduced a system of payment by results (PbR). This was designed to ensure that money flowed with patients as:

- PCTs commissioned from a range of providers on the basis of a standard pre-set national tariff, which reflected the complexities of the cases commissioned (the 'casemix')
- instead of block contracts (where service providers were paid a fixed amount for an agreed volume of services in a year), hospitals (and other providers) were paid for the actual activity they undertook.

The main driver behind this initiative was patient choice – by introducing standard tariffs, the need for local negotiation on price was removed and instead the focus was shifted to quality and responsiveness, the things that are important to the patient. The combination of patient choice and PbR was expected to drive an increase in healthcare capacity and deliver shorter patient waiting times.

Both patient choice and PbR were phased in over a period of years. Key milestones in the development of patient choice included:

- providing patients waiting for elective surgery for over six months with the choice of an alternative provider (summer 2004)
- patients requiring a routine elective referral offered a choice of four or five providers (including one private sector provider) at the point of referral (i.e. at their GP) by the end of December 2005
- patients needing to see a specialist able to choose to go to any hospital in England, including many private and independent sector hospitals (from April 2008).

The first steps to introduce the new PbR financial framework were taken in 2003/04 with the scope extended progressively since then. Chapter 18 looks in more detail at PbR.

NHS foundation trusts

NHS foundation trusts (FTs) were created as new legal entities in the form of public benefit corporations by the *Health and Social Care (Community Health and Standards) Act 2003* – now consolidated in the *NHS Act 2006*. They were introduced to help implement the Labour Government's 10-year *NHS Plan* – by creating a new form of NHS trust that had greater freedoms and more extensive powers, it was hoped that services would improve more quickly.

Initially, applications for foundation status were restricted to a number of 'three-star' trusts with the first wave of FTs coming into being in April 2004. Since then there has been a steady growth in the number of FTs although the pace slowed as organisations struggled to demonstrate their long-term financial viability in the light of difficult economic circumstances, and increased expectations in relation to efficiency. The application process for FT status also changed with an increased focus on clinical quality in the light of high profile governance failures, such as that at Mid-Staffordshire NHS Foundation Trust.

As part of its reform programme, the Coalition Government expects all remaining NHS trusts to achieve foundation status as swiftly as possible – however there is no longer a 'blanket deadline'.

Commissioning a Patient-led NHS, 2005

Following a consultation process in 2005, a reconfiguration of SHAs, PCTs and ambulance trusts was launched by the Department of Health with a significant reduction in their overall numbers. The aim was to reduce management overheads and generate cost savings that could be re-invested in the provision of healthcare.

The reduction in PCT numbers was consistent with the simplification of the commissioning process inherent in the patient choice and PbR initiatives. Increasingly patients were able to select their preferred healthcare provider, thereby refocusing the commissioning role on assessing overall supply levels, negotiating provider standards, and managing demand.

SHAs also reduced from 28 to 10 to reflect the geographical span of the government offices for the regions, and so make working with other public sector partners easier.

Ambulance trust merger was designed to achieve purchasing and management economies of scale and to allow them to develop greater resilience than was possible with smaller scale operations.

Practice based commissioning

Practice based commissioning (PBC) was introduced in 2005/06 with a view to enabling primary care clinicians to take commissioning decisions themselves, thereby providing patients with higher quality services that better suited their needs and circumstances. The underlying presumption was that primary care professionals were in the best position to decide what services their patients needed and to redesign them accordingly. Unlike GP fund holding, which was a feature of the original purchaser/provider split of the 1990s, PBC covered both emergency services and elective activity.

Under PBC, responsibility for commissioning along with an associated budget from the PCT was allocated to some primary care clinicians. However, because PCTs remained legally responsible for managing the money and negotiating and managing all contracts with providers, the budget was notional or 'indicative'. In practice this meant that although primary care clinicians determined the range of services to be provided for their population, the PCT acted as their agent to undertake any required procurements and to carry out the administrative tasks that underpinned these processes.

The Darzi Review – High Quality Care for All, 2007

In July 2007, the Government asked the then health minister Lord Darzi to carry out a wide ranging review of the NHS. An interim report was issued in October 2007 and recommended a number of changes to the provision of healthcare services within the primary and secondary care sectors, including the development of 'poly-clinics' where appropriate – a primary healthcare equivalent of the 'one-stop shop'. The final report – High Quality Care for All – was issued in June 2008 (in time for the 60th anniversary of the NHS on 5th July 2008) and set out a vision of an NHS that 'gives patients and the public more information and choice, works in partnership and has quality of care at its heart'.

The NHS Constitution, 2010

In January 2010, the first ever NHS Constitution came into effect with all providers and commissioners of NHS care now under a statutory duty to have regard to the Constitution in all their decisions and actions. As the Department of Health's website states: 'This means that the Constitution, its pledges, principles, values and responsibilities need to be fully embedded and ingrained into everything the NHS does.'

Equity and Excellence: Liberating the NHS, 2010 and the Health and Social Care Act, 2012

In July 2010, following the formation of the Coalition Government, the Secretary of State for Health issued a series of consultation papers that signalled far-reaching changes for the NHS in England. These proposals (amended in places) were enacted in the Health and Social Care Act 2012 resulting in a new structure and approach for the NHS from April 2013.

The NHS now

The structure introduced by the 2012 Act is shown in the diagram below and came into effect in April 2013:

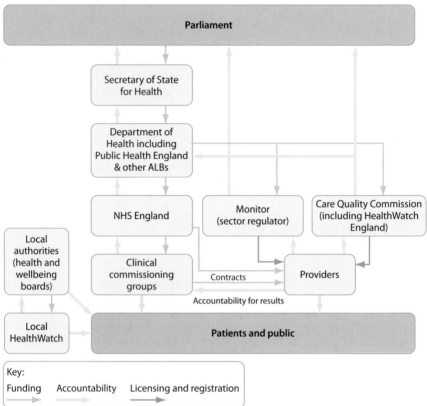

NHS Structure from April 2013

The roles and responsibilities of all the key players are discussed in later chapters of this Guide but in summary the key changes introduced by the 2012 Act are:

Key Changes Introduced by the 2012 Act

- Abolishing SHAs and PCTs from April 2013
- Introducing NHS England to authorise clinical commissioning groups (CCGs), allocate funding to them and commission some services itself
- Handing the majority of NHS commissioning to CCGs that are authorised by (and accountable to) NHS England
- Extending Monitor's role to that of sector regulator for the health and social care sectors with responsibility for licensing healthcare providers, setting and regulating prices and (with NHS England) ensuring continuity of services

- Strengthening the role of the Care Quality Commission (CQC)
- Setting up the NHS Trust Development Authority within the Department of Health to oversee NHS trusts and support the FT 'pipeline'
- Introducing more best practice tariffs 'so that providers are paid according to the costs of excellent care rather than average price'
- Allowing commissioners to pay quality increments and impose contractual penalties
- Continuing QIPP (quality, innovation, productivity and prevention) with a 'stronger focus on general practice leadership'
- Giving FTs greater freedom on income, governance and mergers
- Handing responsibility for public health (with an associated ring fenced budget) to local authorities with Public Health England set up within the Department of Health
- Setting up 'health and wellbeing boards' in every upper tier local authority to 'join up commissioning across the NHS, social care, public health and other services ... directly related to health and wellbeing'
- Developing local HealthWatch organisations from existing local involvement networks to ensure that the views of patients, carers and the public are taken into account
- Setting up HealthWatch England as an independent committee within the CQC to support and lead local HealthWatch.

References and Further Reading

The New NHS: Modern, Dependable (1997 White Paper) – Department of Health archived web pages: www.archive.official-documents.co.uk/document/doh/newnhs/forward.htm

1999 Health Act: www.legislation.gov.uk/ukpga/1999/8/section/60

Care Quality Commission: www.cqc.org.uk/

National Institute for Health and Care Excellence (NICE): www.nice.org.uk

NHS Shared Business Services: www.sbs.nhs.uk/

NHS Act 2006: www.legislation.gov.uk/ukpga/2006/41/contents

The NHS Plan: a Plan for Investment, a Plan for Reform, Department of Health, 2000 (archived web pages): http://webarchive.nationalarchives.gov.uk/+/www.dh.gov.uk/en/publicationsandstatistics/publications/publicationspolicyandguidance/dh_4002960

Shifting the Balance of Power, Department of Health, 2001 (archived web pages): http://webarchive.nationalarchives.gov.uk/+/www.dh.gov.uk/en/publicationsandstatistics/publications/publicationspolicyandguidance/dh_4009844

Health and Social (Community Standards) Act 2003: www.legislation.gov.uk/ukpga/2003/43/contents

HM Treasury – Comprehensive Spending Reviews and Budget Reports: www.hm-treasury.gov.uk/spend_index.htm

Quality, innovation, productivity and prevention (QIPP), Department of Health: https://www.gov.uk/government/policies/making-the-nhs-more-efficient-and-less-bureaucratic

Delivering the NHS Improvement Plan, Department of Health, 2002 (archived web pages): http://webarchive.nationalarchives.gov.uk/+/www.dh.gov.uk/en/publicationsandstatistics/publications/annualreports/browsable/DH_5277178

Payment by Results: https://www.gov.uk/government/publications/payment-by-results-pbr-operational-guidance-and-tariffs

Commissioning a Patient-led NHS, Department of Health, 2005 (archived web pages): http://webarchive.nationalarchives.gov.uk/+/www.dh.gov.uk/en/Managingyourorganisation/Commissioning/CommissioningapatientledNHS/index.htm

Practice Based Commissioning – Department of Health (archived web pages): http://webarchive.nationalarchives.gov.uk/+/www.dh.gov.uk/en/Managingyourorganisation/Commissioning/Practice-basedcommissioning/index.htm

Our NHS Our Future: NHS Next Stage Review (the Darzi review), 2007: http://www.nhshistory.net/darzi-interim.pdf

High Quality Care for all: NHS Next Stage Review final report, Department of Health, 2008 (archived web pages): http://webarchive.nationalarchives.gov.uk/+/www.dh.gov.uk/en/Publicationsandstatistics/Publications/PublicationsPolicyandGuidance/DH_085825

The NHS Constitution for England, Department of Health, 2013: https://www.gov.uk/government/publications/the-nhs-constitution-for-england

Equity and Excellence: Liberating the NHS (and associated consultation papers), Department of Health, 2010: https://www.gov.uk/government/publications/liberating-the-nhs-white-paper

Chapter 3: NHS Finance – Who Does What?

The Role of Government, Ministers, the Department of Health (including its ALBs) and NHS Property Services Ltd

> Overview
>
> This chapter focuses on the role of the 'centre' in relation to NHS finance and governance – we will look in turn at:
>
> * Parliament
> * Government ministers
> * the Department of Health and its associated arm's length bodies (ALBs)
> * the NHS Trust Development Authority
> * Public Health England
> * Health Education England
> * NHS Property Services limited.
>
> For each element, the chapter looks at its status; accountabilities; roles and financing. To remind yourself of the overall structure of the NHS and where 'the centre' fits, look back at the diagram on page 16.

Parliament

What it is – status and accountabilities

Parliament is the highest legislative body in the land and so sits at the top of the 'accountability tree'. In relation to the NHS, Parliament holds the Secretary of State for Health to account for its functioning and use of resources.

What Parliament does – roles and responsibilities

As well as holding the Secretary of State to account, the cross party House of Commons Health Committee examines the expenditure, administration and policy of the Department of Health and its associated bodies. The members of this committee are appointed by the House of Commons and its constitution and powers are set out in *House of Commons Standing Order No.152.*

The Health Committee has a maximum of eleven members and the quorum for any formal proceedings is three. As the members of the committee are appointed by the House they remain on the committee until the next dissolution of Parliament, unless discharged.

Within its remit, the committee has complete discretion to decide which areas to investigate and has the power to require the submission of written evidence and documents, and to send for and examine witnesses. The committee's oral evidence sessions are usually open to the public and are often televised. Deliberative meetings are held in private.

When an inquiry ends, a report is agreed by the committee and then published by Her Majesty's Stationery Office. The report is usually published in two volumes: the findings of the committee and the background (memoranda and oral) evidence. The Government is committed to responding to such reports within two months of publication.

The committee is supported in its work by a team of staff and by part-time specialists, usually academics or experts from professions relevant to its inquiries.

Two other Parliamentary committees scrutinise the Department of Health and the health service:

- the Public Accounts Committee (PAC)
- the Public Administration Select Committee (PASC).

The PAC keeps a check on all public expenditure including money spent on health. Its remit takes it far wider than a view on the annual accounts, with the results of National Audit Office value for money studies usually being considered. In these instances, the PAC takes evidence, usually questioning key senior managers from relevant organisations (such as the Department of Health, Monitor and NHS England), before publishing its own report and making recommendations.

The PASC examines the reports of the Parliamentary and Health Service Ombudsmen and considers matters relating to the quality and standards of civil service administration.

Other select committees may from time to time conduct inquiries into Government policies that impact upon the Department of Health.

How Parliament is financed

Parliament is funded by public money (i.e. by taxpayers).

Secretary of State for Health

What the role is – status and accountabilities

The Secretary of State for Health is a Cabinet minister with 'ultimate responsibility for ensuring the whole [health and care] system works together to meet the needs of patients and the public and reflect their experiences'.[1] The Secretary of State is accountable to Parliament.

What the Secretary of State does – roles and responsibilities

The NHS was established under the *National Health Service Act 1946*. This and other subsequent Acts of Parliament relating to the NHS set out the duty of the Secretary of State for Health to provide a comprehensive health service in England.

---

[1] *The Health and Care System Explained*, March 2013, gov.uk website.

The Secretary of State is politically accountable for the NHS and for the resources allocated to the health and social care system and also has a duty to 'maximise the autonomy' of commissioners and providers by 'limiting his general powers of direction'.

He or she is also responsible for:

- system design
- the legislative framework
- overall strategic direction
- progress against national outcomes.

Health Ministers

What they are – status and accountabilities

The Secretary of State is supported by a team of health ministers who are appointed by the Government. These ministers are either MPs elected by the public, or members of the House of Lords. They are accountable to the Secretary of State.

What ministers do – roles and responsibilities

Health ministers each have individual responsibility for different aspects of the Department of Health's work. The portfolios attached to the ministerial posts often change, depending on the priorities at that point in time and the personal interests of the individuals. For the latest information on ministerial portfolios see the Department's website.

The Department of Health

What it is – status and accountabilities

The Department of Health is the Department of State responsible for the NHS, public health and adult social care in England and is accountable via its 'Principal Accounting Officer' (the permanent secretary) to Parliament 'for the proper use of the resources allocated to the Department'.[2]

The Department supports the Secretary of State and ministers in carrying out their ministerial responsibilities including:

- accounting to Parliament and the public for the way money is spent and what is achieved with it
- answering Parliamentary questions and dealing with other Parliamentary business such as debates and enquiries
- responding to communications from the public and MPs
- communicating with the public.

---

[2] *Accounting Officer System Statement*, Department of Health, August 2012.

There is a Departmental Board chaired by the Secretary of State which includes non-executives from outside Government. This Board 'scrutinises reports on performance, and challenges the Department on how well it is achieving its objectives'.[3]

To give you an idea of the Department's size, it employs around 2,300 people, with headquarters staff based in Leeds and London. This staffing level is expected to decrease to 1,700 over the next few years.

What the Department of Health does – roles and responsibilities

The Department's website states that its overarching purpose is to help people to live better for longer by leading, shaping and funding health and care in England, 'making sure people have the support, care and treatment they need, with the compassion, respect and dignity they deserve'. The website identifies the Department's responsibilities as being to:

- create national policies and legislation, providing the long-term vision and ambition to meet current and future challenges, putting health and care at the heart of Government, and being a global leader in health and care policy
- support the integrity of the health and care system by providing funding, assuring the delivery and continuity of services, and accounting to Parliament in a way that represents the best interests of the patient, public and taxpayer
- champion innovation and improvement by supporting research and technology, promoting honesty, openness and transparency, and instilling an organisational culture that values compassion, dignity and the highest quality of care above everything.

The Department of Health's website also lists five key priorities.

> **The Department's Priorities – 2012 and 2013**
>
> 1. Making sure patients and the public are at the heart of the health and care system
> 2. Improving the nation's health through better health services
> 3. Making the health and care system more accountable
> 4. Improving public health
> 5. Reforming long-term and social care.

Linked to these responsibilities and priorities, the Department has a number of key roles including:

- providing leadership for the NHS, adult social care and public health services (including for example, health promotion, health protection against infectious diseases, the safety of medicines and ethical issues) and setting the strategic framework within which they operate
- developing policy and legislation relating to the NHS, adult social care and public health
- supporting the delivery of improvements in the health and adult social care system via performance monitoring and evaluation; managerial and professional leadership of external groups; building capacity and capability and ensuring value for money

---

[3] *Accounting Officer System Statement*, Department of Health, August 2012.

- leading on the integration of health and wellbeing into wider Government policy
- allocating the funding received from the Treasury
- setting healthcare standards, targets and outcome measures – there are separate 'outcomes frameworks' for the NHS, public health and adult social care
- agreeing an annual mandate with NHS England based on these outcomes frameworks
- reviewing the performance of its arm's length bodies (see below)and intervening (by direction) if necessary
- managing performance against its statutory responsibilities and holding the NHS to account – this includes ensuring that the NHS lives within its allocated resources and achieves required efficiency savings (£20bn by 2015).

These roles are translated into a number of specific 'deliverables' for the NHS by NHS England which is responsible for the day-to-day operational management of the NHS and operates at arm's length from the Department (see chapter 4).

How the Department of Health is financed

The Treasury sets the Department of Health's budget for a three-year period in a budgetary exercise known as the spending review, which takes place across Government. The Department submits evidence to the Treasury setting out its proposals for expenditure plans covering the three-year period. These plans are then discussed and challenged over several months before being finalised. The outcome of the most recent spending review was released in October 2010 and covers the years 2011/12 to 2014/15. The results of the next spending review are due to be announced in June 2013.

Once the Treasury has set the overall budget total, the Department determines how this should be allocated. The vast majority of funding is allocated to NHS England but some is retained in central budgets. For example, for 2013/14, the total revenue budget for the NHS is around £106.9 billion of which £95.6 billion is allocated to NHS England. The Department of Health's funding also finances the NHS Trust Development Authority (NHS TDA); Public Health England (PHE) and its other associated arm's length bodies (ALBs) (see below).

Once resources have been allocated, the Department of Health has an on-going responsibility to ensure that the NHS lives within them, and that its objectives are achieved as efficiently as possible. This includes monitoring performance against national targets.

Arm's Length Bodies

What they are – status and accountabilities

Arm's length bodies (ALBs) are stand-alone national organisations sponsored by the Department of Health to undertake activities to help deliver its agenda. They range in size but tend to have Boards, employ staff and publish accounts. In constitutional terms, there are three types of ALB.[4]

---

[4] The Department of Health also works with a number of 'advisory non-departmental bodies' such as the NHS Pay Review Body and the Advisory Committee on Clinical Excellence Awards.

Types of ALB

Executive agencies – these are part of the Department (and are accountable to it) but have greater operational independence than a division or section of the Department.

Special health authorities – these are independent bodies (although they are subject to ministerial direction) that are created by order.

Executive non-departmental public bodies (ENDPBs) – these are established by primary legislation and have their own statutory functions. Their relationship with the Department is defined in legislation and some have greater independence than others. They all play important roles but are not part of the Department.

Regardless of their status, every ALB has a 'framework agreement' which sets out its relationship with the Department – in particular, these agreements cover:

- lines of accountability
- working arrangements
- core financial requirements
- relationships with other ALBs and organisations in the system
- how the ALB is held to account for delivering its objectives and outcomes and for the use of public money.

Each ALB must also submit a business plan to the Department for approval each year indicating how its objectives will be achieved and forecasting its financial performance. Every ALB must lay its annual report and accounts before Parliament.

The Department has a duty to keep the performance of ALBs under review and the Secretary of State can intervene in the event of 'significant failure'.

What ALBs do – roles and responsibilities

ALBs can be categorised by function as follows – we will look more closely at those that have a particular bearing on NHS finance and governance later in this chapter.

ALBs Categorised by Function

Regulatory – ALBs that hold the health and social care system to account:

NHS England (ENDPB)
Care Quality Commission (ENDPB)
Human Fertilisation and Embryology Authority (ENDPB – until 2015)
Human Tissue Authority (ENDPB – until 2015)
Medicines and Healthcare Products Regulatory Agency (executive agency)
Monitor (ENDPB)
NHS Trust Development Authority (special health authority).

Public welfare – ALBs that focus primarily on safety and the protection of public and patients:

Public Health England (executive agency)
Health Research Authority (special health authority).

Standards – ALBs that focus primarily on establishing national standards and best practice:

National Institute for Health and Care Excellence (NICE) (from April 2013, an ENDPB – prior to the 2012 Act it was a special health authority).

Central services to the NHS – ALBs that provide cost-effective services and focused expertise across the health and social care system:

NHS Business Services Authority (special health authority)
Health Education England (special health authority)
Health and Social Care Information Centre (ENDPB)
NHS Blood and Transplant (special health authority)
NHS Litigation Authority (special health authority).

How ALBs are financed

ALBs are financed primarily out of the settlement received by the Department of Health (as 'grant in aid') although some levy fees for services provided (for example, the CQC charges a registration fee) and others charge users of their services – for example, in the case of NHS Blood and Transplant, hospitals (both NHS and private) pay for each unit of blood supplied.

NHS Trust Development Authority (NHS TDA)

What it is – status and accountabilities

The NHS TDA was established by the 2012 Act as a time limited special health authority. It is located within the Department of Health and has teams in London and Leeds with a staff of around 150. It is an independent body within the Department of Health but is accountable to it and subject to ministerial direction.

What the NHS TDA does – roles and responsibilities

The NHS TDA is responsible for overseeing all remaining NHS trusts and for supporting them (including providing tailored support to each trust) as they move towards foundation status. The Government wants this to happen as soon as possible, although there is now no blanket deadline – instead each trust has its own target date. The intention is that once all trusts are foundations, the NHS TDA will be wound up.

The NHS TDA also has responsibility for:

- public appointments for NHS trusts (Chairperson and non-executive directors) and some trustee appointments for NHS charities
- the designation of 'Accountable Officers'[5] for NHS trusts
- advising the Secretary of State as to whether or not a trust should be placed into the failure regime
- overseeing NHS trusts via annual plans, performance agreements, monitoring and performance management
- assessing mergers and acquisitions of NHS trusts by other NHS or foundation trusts
- approving capital investments or significant commercial transactions by NHS trusts (see chapter 15 for more about delegated limits for capital spending).

How the NHS TDA is financed

The NHS TDA is funded via the Department of Health's allocation.

Public Health England

What it is – status and accountabilities

As we have seen earlier in this chapter, the Department of Health has overall responsibility for setting the policy and legal framework in relation to public health. To help it discharge this responsibility a new organisation – Public Health England – was established under the 2012 Act as an executive agency of the Department of Health. This means that PHE is accountable to the Department.

PHE employs 5,500 staff, most of whom are scientists, researchers and public health professionals. It is organised into 4 regions and 15 local centres.

What PHE does – roles and responsibilities

PHE's role is to protect and improve the health and wellbeing of the population and reduce health inequalities. In particular, it is responsible at a national level for 'preparing, planning and responding to emergencies and health protection incidents'.[6] It does this by working closely with the health and social care system and other public services. Although PHE provides leadership, local authorities are responsible for health improvement and reducing health inequalities at local level (see chapter 8).

Healthy Lives, Healthy People: Update on Public Health Funding identified three elements to PHE's role:

- delivering services such as public health information and intelligence
- leading on public health by building relationships and encouraging accountability and transparency
- supporting the development of the public health workforce by appointing (with local authorities) Directors of Public Health and supporting excellence in public health practice.

---

[5] Every NHS organisation must have an 'Accountable Officer' – see chapter 13 for more details.
[6] *Accounting Officer System Statement*, Department of Health.

PHE's website lists its responsibilities as being:

- making the public healthier by encouraging discussions, advising Government and supporting action by local government, the NHS and other people and organisations
- supporting the public so they can protect and improve their own health
- protecting the nation's health through the national health protection service, and preparing for public health emergencies
- sharing our information and expertise with local authorities, industry and the NHS, to help them make improvements in the public's health
- researching, collecting and analysing data to improve our understanding of health and come up with answers to public health problems
- reporting on improvements in the public's health so everyone can understand the challenge and the next steps
- helping local authorities and the NHS to develop the public health system and its specialist workforce.

How PHE is financed

PHE is financed out of the Department of Health's allocation.

Health Education England

What it is – status and accountabilities

Health Education England (HEE) was established by the 2012 Act as a special health authority within the Department of Health. It is located in Leeds (with a small office in London) and has between 120 and 150 staff. In due course the intention is for the HEE to be established in primary legislation as an ENDPB.

What HEE does – roles and responsibilities

HEE provides 'national leadership and oversight on strategic planning and development of the health and public health workforce' and allocates education and training resources. In other words, HEE ensures that the healthcare workforce has the right skills and is available in the right numbers.

Instead of continuing with the range of different funding sources that existed prior to April 2013 (for example, for multi-professional education and training (MPET) and the service increment for teaching (SIFT) to support the additional costs incurred in providing clinical placements for medical undergraduates), HEE intends to operate a single budget.

One other key area that HEE is responsible for is working with 'Local Education and Training Boards' (LETBs) to improve the quality of education and training outcomes so that they meet the needs of providers, the public and patients. LETBs are statutory committees of HEE. They are based in local offices and have taken on the workforce planning and education and training functions previously carried out by strategic health authorities. There are thirteen LETBs which are accountable to HEE.

How HEE is financed

HEE is financed out of the Department of Health's allocation.

NHS Property Services Ltd

What it is – status and accountabilities

NHS Property Services Limited was set up in 2012 to take over the residual estate left by strategic health authorities and primary care trusts (PCTs) after their abolition. In terms of its constitution, it is a company wholly owned by the Government and is also known as PropCo. It has 3,000 staff, most of whom have transferred to it from the abolished organisations.

What it does – roles and responsibilities

NHS Property Services Limited's role is to maintain, manage and develop around 3,600 NHS facilities. Its objectives are 'to:

- hold property for use by community and primary care services, including for use by social enterprises
- deliver value for money property services
- cut costs of administering the estate by consolidating the management of over 150 estates
- deliver and develop cost-effective property solutions for community health services
- dispose of property surplus to NHS requirements.'[7]

The company has taken on 'existing contractual arrangements with service providers that deliver and maintain NHS properties'. It operates on a local basis and is coterminous with local NHS organisations.

In practice this involves NHS Property Services Ltd in delivering a range of services classified as 'core' (such as property management advice and strategic estate management) across England. 'Additional services' (such as cleaning, catering and grounds maintenance) are also offered where they had previously been provided by PCTs. There are a number of other services that the company has specifically said it will not provide – these include telephony and the management of transport.

How NHS Property Services Ltd is financed

Although NHS Property Services is a company, it is 'wholly owned by the Secretary of State for Health'[8] and is financed from the Department's allocation.

---

[7] *Written Ministerial Statement*, Department of Health, January 2012:
www.parliament.uk/documents/commons-vote-office/2.Health-NHS-property-services.pdf.

[8] NHS Property Services Letter to the System, November 2012.

References and Further Reading

For details of legislation including Health Acts: www.legislation.gov.uk/

Select Committees: www.parliament.uk/business/committees/

The Health and Care System Explained, March 2013: www.gov.uk/government/publications/the-health-and-care-system-explained/the-health-and-care-system-explained

Department of Health website – for details of how the Department works and ministerial roles: www.gov.uk/government/organisations/department-of-health

Accounting Officer System Statement, Department of Health, August 2012: https://www.gov.uk/government/uploads/system/uploads/attachment_data/file/126966/Accounting-Officer-system-statement.pdf.pdf

Spending reviews and budgets – details available from the treasury's website: www.hm-treasury.gov.uk/spend_index.htm

Department of Health Arm's Length Bodies (includes links to all those referred to in the chapter): www.gov.uk/government/organisations#department-of-health

NHS Trust Development Authority: www.ntda.nhs.uk/

Public Health England: https://www.gov.uk/government/organisations/public-health-england

Health Education England: http://hee.nhs.uk/

Our Strategic Intent, HEE, 2013: http://hee.nhs.uk/2013/01/31/our-strategic-intent/

NHS Property Services Ltd: www.property.nhs.uk/

Written Ministerial Statement on NHS Property Services Ltd, Department of Health, January 2012: www.parliament.uk/documents/commons-vote-office/2.Health-NHS-property-services.pdf

NHS Property Services Ltd Letter to the System, November 2012: www.property.nhs.uk/nhs-property-services-ltd-letter-to-the-system/

Chapter 4: NHS Finance – Who Does What?

The Role of NHS England

> ### Overview
>
> This chapter looks what NHS England is, how it is structured and the role it plays in relation to NHS finance and governance. To remind yourself of where NHS England fits into the NHS structure, look back at the diagram on page 16.

What is NHS England?

NHS England was set up under section 9 of the *Health and Social Care Act 2012* and became fully operational on 1st April 2013. Until March 2013 it was called the NHS Commissioning Board.

In constitutional terms, NHS England is an executive non-departmental body working at arm's length from the Department of Health (i.e. it is a Department of Health arm's length body or ALB). NHS England has a Board, central department, 4 regions, 27 area teams (also referred to as 'local area teams') and 12 clinical senates. The area teams act as local offices of NHS England, with functions that include commissioning primary care services. Ten of the area teams have been designated as 'hubs' for specialised commissioning, while a smaller number commission prison and military health. NHS England's headquarters are in Leeds but it also has a London office. Although it has a regional and local presence, NHS England's website makes it clear that it is 'one single organisation operating to a common model with one Board'.

NHS England is accountable to the Secretary of State for Health and the Department of Health for meeting its legal duties and fulfilling its 'mandate'. In formal terms, the line of accountability runs from NHS England's Accounting Officer (the Chief Executive, as designated in the 2012 Act) to the Secretary of State (through the Department of Health) and Parliament.

The mandate is a multi-year document that is updated and published each year. It sets out the objectives that NHS England is expected to deliver in the forthcoming year along with its financial allocation. In response to the mandate, NHS England publishes an annual business plan that shows how it will achieve the objectives it has been set and an annual report showing how it performed.

As with all ALBs, there is also a 'framework agreement' that sets out the working relationship and lines of accountability between the Department and NHS England along with financial requirements and relationships with other organisations (see chapter 3 for more about ALBs).

NHS England is accountable to the Department for staying within its allocated resources (the 'commissioning revenue limit' allocated to it by the Department) as well as delivering a wide range of improvements to healthcare through a number of 'outcomes frameworks'. NHS

England is also responsible for the functioning of the entire commissioning system and the associated budget and for reporting the consolidated financial position of itself and clinical commissioning groups (CCGs).

What NHS England does – Roles and Responsibilities

Alongside the Secretary of State, NHS England has an overriding statutory responsibility for promoting a comprehensive health service that will 'secure improvements in the physical and mental health of the people of England and in the prevention, diagnosis and treatment of physical and mental illness'.[1] As well as general duties (for example, having regard to the NHS Constitution; exercising its functions economically, efficiently and effectively; securing continuous improvement and promoting innovation), NHS England has a number of specific statutory duties relating to:

- establishing and holding CCGs to account (for example, ensuring that there is a comprehensive system of CCGs in place and that each GP practice is a member of a CCG; authorising CCGs)
- commissioning of services (for example, NHS England must commission directly those services specified in regulations – see below)
- partnership working/co-operation (for example, a duty to co-operate with the Department, Monitor, the Care Quality Commission (CQC), the National Institute for Care and Excellence (NICE) and the Health and Social Care Information Centre; meeting safeguarding duties for children and vulnerable groups)
- emergencies – to ensure that it and CCGs are properly prepared and resilient
- finance – to manage overall expenditure on commissioning and administration and produce accounts that include the consolidated accounts of all CCGs.

NHS England allocates funding to CCGs and holds them to account for the management of these public funds. It is also responsible for managing financial risk across CCGs.

As mentioned above, NHS England commissions some services itself (referred to as 'direct commissioning') – specifically:

- primary care services provided by GPs, dentists, opticians and community pharmacists (until April 2013 these were commissioned by primary care trusts)
- specialised services – these account for around 10% or £11.8bn of the annual NHS budget and are defined on NHS England's website as 'those services provided in relatively few hospitals, accessed by comparatively small numbers of patients, but with catchment populations of more than one million. These services tend to be located in specialist hospital trusts that can recruit staff with the appropriate expertise and enable them to develop their skills'. A good example is transplant surgery
- offender healthcare (which includes high security psychiatric facilities)
- some services for members of the armed forces.

---

[1] NHS England's legal duties and powers are set out in sections 9 and 23 and schedule A1 of the 2012 Act.

These services are commissioned by the relevant area team using common 'single operating models' and reporting to a single Board within NHS England. These models have been designed to ensure that all patients are offered consistent, accessible, high quality services across the country.

In addition, although Public Health England (PHE) and local authorities are responsible for commissioning public health services, NHS England commissions many of the public health services delivered by the NHS on their behalf. NHS England has also developed a commissioning model with stakeholders for the £2.2 billion of preventive public health services it commissions directly, namely:

- the national immunisation programmes
- the national screening programmes
- public health services for offenders in custody
- sexual assault referral centres
- public health services for children aged 0–5 years
- child health information systems.

In total NHS England's direct commissioning activities account for £20bn and involve NHS England in holding around 35,000 contracts for primary care services. NHS England 'performance manages' these contracts – not CCGs.

NHS England is also required to carry out a number of other roles, including those set out below:

NHS England's 'other' Roles

- Setting commissioning guidelines
- Developing model care pathways
- Establishing model contracts for commissioning groups to use when commissioning services
- Supporting CCGs as they develop their skills and capacity
- Determining the structure of future payment systems (i.e. for payment by results)
- Promoting and extending choice
- The roll-out of personal health budgets
- Championing patient and carer involvement
- Hosting 'clinical senates' (doctors, nurses and other professionals who advise NHS England, CCGs and health and wellbeing boards on 'strategic clinical decision making to support commissioners') and clinical networks (to advise on specific areas of care such as cancer)
- Overseeing the cancer drugs fund

Commissioning support units

NHS England also hosts commissioning support units (CSUs) for which a hosting charge is levied. CSUs have grown out of primary care trusts and provide non-clinical support and services to CCGs, helping them to deliver their commissioning role. This may be in the form of back office functions such as finance (for which, there is a new 'integrated single financial environment' that CCGs, CSUs and NHS England must use) and human resources; providing data analysis and storage; developing the health needs assessment or handling media enquiries.

Arrangements between CSUs and CCGs are covered by service level agreements (SLAs) that set out the expectations and requirements of each party. NHS England has set out in guidance 'key minimum clauses' that it would expect to see in these SLAs along with an example agreement and template.

Each CSU is led by a managing director and operates with a governing body (but not a legal Board) – as they are part of NHS England, all hosted CSUs fall within NHS England's own governance arrangements.

CSUs operate under a licence granted by NHS England and are required to break even with any profits reinvested into the business. The licence includes the powers delegated by NHS England and reflects any additional conditions under which the CSU must operate.

NHS England will host CSUs until they become independent organisations. The intention is that this will happen by 2016.

Area teams

There are 27 area teams – 9 in the north; 8 in the midlands and east; 7 in the south and 3 in London. Their core functions are focussed on:

- CCG development and assurance
- emergency planning, resilience and response
- quality and safety
- partnerships
- configuration
- system oversight.

As mentioned earlier, these area teams also commission GP, dental and pharmacy services and certain aspects of optical services. Ten of the teams act as specialised commissioning hubs with a smaller number commissioning military and offender health services.

Area teams are supported by local professional networks (LPNs) that work in partnership with CCGs to help provide clinical leadership and support the implementation of national strategies and policies at local level. See NHS England's guide *Securing Excellence in Commissioning Primary Care* for more details.

Clinical senates and networks

As mentioned earlier, NHS England hosts 12 clinical senates, aligned largely with area team and specialised commissioning hub boundaries. Their role is to help CCGs, health and wellbeing boards and NHS England to make the best possible decisions about healthcare for the population they serve.

There are also a number of clinical networks that are also hosted by NHS England – these advise on specific areas of care such as cancer.

How NHS England is Financed

NHS England's budget is allocated to it by the Department of Health. Most of this budget is then allocated to CCGs and used by them to commission services. To give you an idea of the amount of money involved, the total revenue budget that NHS England oversees in 2013/14 is £95.6bn with £64.7bn of this allocated to CCGs (this includes £1.3bn for CCG running costs). NHS England's own running costs amount to around £527m and its direct commissioning (excluding that carried out for public health) accounts for £25.4bn. See chapter 10 for more details and a full breakdown of the 2013/14 budget.

NHS England also has a capital budget for 2013/14 of £200m.

References and Further Reading

Health and Social Care Act 2012: www.legislation.gov.uk/ukpga/2012/7/contents/enacted

NHS England: www.england.nhs.uk/

NHS Mandate, 2012: http://mandate.dh.gov.uk/

Putting Patients Frist: the NHS England business plan for 2013/14 – 2015/16: www.england.nhs.uk/wp-content/uploads/2013/04/ppf-1314–1516.pdf

NHS England Operating Models for direct commissioning: www.england.nhs.uk/resources/d-com/

Clinical Senates and Networks: www.england.nhs.uk/resources/networks-senates/Information about personal health budgets: www.personalhealthbudgets.england.nhs.uk/

SLAs for CCGs and CSUs – see the CCG resources page of NHS England's website: www.england.nhs.uk/resources/resources-for-ccgs/

Information about the Integrated Single Financial Environment: www.england.nhs.uk/resources/resources-for-ccgs/isfe/

NHS Outcomes Framework 2013/14: www.gov.uk/government/publications/nhs-outcomes-framework-2013-to-2014

Securing Excellence in Commissioning Primary Care, NHS England, June 2012: www.england.nhs.uk/wp-content/uploads/2012/06/ex-comm-pc.pdf

Chapter 5: NHS finance – Who Does What?

The Role of Clinical Commissioning Groups

> **Overview**
>
> This chapter looks at what clinical commissioning groups (CCGs) are, how they are structured and what they do with a focus on accountability, governance and finance. To remind yourself of where CCGs sit in the NHS structure, look back at the diagram on page 16.

What are CCGs?

Constitution

CCGs are new statutory bodies created by the *Health and Social Care Act 2012* that cover the whole of England. They came into existence in shadow form during 2011/12 and took over their statutory roles from 1st April 2013.

Every CCG must be authorised by NHS England. This authorisation process is designed to confirm that a CCG can:

- 'commission safely
- use its budget responsibly
- exercise its functions to improve quality, reduce inequality and deliver improved outcomes within the available resources.'[1]

It involves an assessment across six domains and in each case thresholds must be met.

> **CCG Authorisation – the Six Domains**
>
> 1. A strong clinical and multi-professional focus which brings real added value.
> 2. Meaningful engagement with patients, carers and their communities.
> 3. Clear and credible plans which continue to deliver the QIPP (quality, innovation, productivity and prevention) challenge within financial resources, in line with national requirements (including outcomes) and local joint health and wellbeing strategies.
> 4. Proper constitutional and governance arrangements, with the capacity and capability to deliver all their duties and responsibilities, including financial control, as well as effectively commission all the services for which they are responsible.
> 5. Collaborative arrangements for commissioning with other CCGs, local authorities and NHS England as well as the appropriate external commissioning support.
> 6. Great leaders who individually and collectively can make a real difference.

---

[1] *CCG Authorisation: Key Facts*, NHS England.

Full details are set out on NHS England's authorisation web pages.

There are 211 CCGs across England covering areas that are largely in line with upper tier or unitary local authority boundaries. Where this is not the case and a CCG straddles more than one local authority it must be for 'patient interest reasons'. Of the 211 CCGs, 106 were 'fully authorised' on 1st April 2013 (i.e. there were no conditions attached) and 14 were 'authorised with legal directions' (i.e. the conditions of their authorisation were underpinned by 'legally-mandated support from NHS England). The remaining 91 were authorised 'with conditions'. These conditions are reviewed regularly and removed once CCGs have 'demonstrated progress'.[2]

Structure

In terms of their structure, each CCG is made up of members that are the GP practices within its area. They have a 'Council of Members' (on which all the constituent GP practices are represented) and **must** also have a governing body, a Chair, an 'Accountable Officer' (see below) and a Chief Finance Officer (CFO). The Council of Members delegates functions to the governing body (or to its members/employees; committees or sub-committees).

NHS England's *Model Constitution* for CCGs states that the governing body is statutorily responsible for:

- 'ensuring that the group has appropriate arrangements in place to exercise its functions effectively, efficiently and economically and in accordance with the group's principles of good governance (its main function)
- determining the remuneration, fees and other allowances payable to employees or other persons providing services to the group and the allowances payable under any pension scheme ...
- approving any functions of the group that are specified in regulations
- other functions delegated to it by the CCG.'

Although the Accountable Officer in a CCG is a senior leadership role, it is not the same as the Chief Executive in other NHS organisations and will often be filled by a clinical leader. It is for the CCG to nominate its Accountable Officer but he or she is formally appointed by NHS England. The role of the Accountable Officer is set out in NHS England guidance[3] as:

- being responsible for ensuring that the CCG fulfils its duties to exercise its functions effectively, efficiently and economically thus ensuring improvement in the quality of services and the health of the local population whilst maintaining value for money
- ensuring that the regularity and propriety of expenditure is discharged at all times, and that arrangements are put in place to ensure that good practice is embodied and that safeguarding of funds is ensured through effective financial and management systems

---

[2] NHS England news release, 27 March 2013: www.england.nhs.uk/2013/03/27/gp-commissioning/.
[3] *Clinical Commissioning Group Governing Body Members: Role Outlines, Attributes and Skills*, NHS England, 2012.

- working closely with the Chair of the governing body, ensuring that proper constitutional, governance and development arrangements are put in place to assure the members (through the governing body) of the organisation's on-going capability and capacity to meet its duties and responsibilities (including arrangements for the on-going development of its members and staff).

In the same guidance, the Chief Finance Officer's role is described as:

- being the governing body's professional expert on finance and ensuring, through robust systems and processes, the regularity and propriety of expenditure is fully discharged
- making appropriate arrangements to support, monitor and report on the CCG's finances
- overseeing robust audit and governance arrangements leading to propriety in the use of the CCG's resources
- being able to advise the governing body on the effective, efficient and economic use of the group's allocation, to remain within that allocation and deliver required financial targets and duties
- producing the financial statements for audit and publication in accordance with the statutory requirements to demonstrate effective stewardship of public money and accountability to NHS England.

Accountabilities

CCGs are accountable to NHS England (for improving outcomes to patients and for getting the best possible value for money from the money they receive) and to the public and patients. The formal accountability link is from the CCG's Accountable Officer to NHS England's Accounting Officer but from the public/patient viewpoint the key document is the CCG's written constitution which is developed as part of the authorisation process. This document is a statutory requirement and must be available to the public.

A CCG's constitution sets out how it will meet its responsibilities and describes its governing principles, rules and procedures. NHS England has issued a model that CCGs can use to develop their constitutions.

CCG Constitution – Suggested Content

- The name/membership and area covered
- Mission, values and aims
- Functions and duties
- Decision making – who can decide what
- Roles and responsibilities – for example, of practice representatives; the Chair and Deputy Chair of the governing body; the Accountable Officer and CFO
- Standards of business conduct including the management of conflicts of interest; declarations and registers of interests and transparency in procurement
- Employer's responsibilities
- Standing orders

As well as being a public document, the constitution must be adhered to by:

- the CCG's member practices
- the CCG's employees
- individuals working on behalf of the CCG
- anyone who is a member of the CCG's governing body or any committees/sub-committees established by the governing body.

Although CCGs do not have to follow the suggested format, their constitutions must meet the requirements set out in the 2012 Act.

CCGs must also adhere to the *Commissioning Outcomes Indicator Set* developed by the National Institute for Care Excellence (NICE) in line with the expectation set out in the mandate agreed between NHS England and the Department of Health (see chapter 3). This provides clear, comparative information about the quality of health services and associated health outcomes. NHS England uses this as part of its ongoing assessment process for CCGs – it looks at performance against the outcomes indicators and also assesses how well CCGs are meeting their financial duties.

If a CCG is unable to fulfil its duties effectively or there is a significant risk of failure, NHS England has powers to intervene. These powers range from telling a CCG how it should discharge its functions through to dissolving a CCG completely if it is failing over a period of time.

What CCGs do – Roles and Responsibilities

CCGs are responsible for agreeing the care that patients registered with their constituent practices need, negotiating contracts with healthcare providers and monitoring their implementation. They commission the majority of NHS services for their patients and are responsible for £64.7 billion of the £95.6 billion NHS commissioning budget.

Services Commissioned by CCGs

- Planned hospital care
- Rehabilitative care
- Maternity services
- Urgent and emergency services including ambulance and out-of-hours services (CCGs must also commission these services for anyone in their area although for some patients the costs will subsequently be charged to the CCG with which they are registered)
- Community health services
- Mental health services
- Learning disabilities services
- Abortion services
- Infertility services
- Continuing healthcare

CCGs are also responsible for managing GP prescribing – they meet the costs of prescriptions written by their member practices but not the associated dispensing fees.

CCGs are **not** responsible for commissioning core primary care (i.e. services provided by GPs, dentists, community pharmacists, and holders of ophthalmic contracts), national and regional specialised services and a number of other prescribed services – these are commissioned by NHS England (see chapter 4).

CCGs must also fulfil a number of other statutory duties which are grouped under four headings in the Department of Health's guide *The Functions of Clinical Commissioning Groups*:

CCG Statutory Duties

General – for example, to co-operate with other NHS bodies; to have regard to the NHS Constitution and guidance on commissioning issued by NHS England; to promote innovation in health service provision; to promote the involvement of patients.

Planning, agreeing, monitoring services – for example, to contribute to the JSNA (joint strategic needs assessment) and JHWS (joint health and wellbeing strategy) and to have regard to them; to prepare and publish a commissioning plan before the start of each financial year which sets out how the CCG will secure improvements in services and outcomes, reduce inequalities, involve patients and fulfil its financial duties; to comply with regulations relating to best practice in procurement/patient choice and anti-competitive conduct.

Finance – for example, to ensure the annual budget, revenue and capital limits and running cost allowance are not exceeded; to provide financial information to NHS England; to keep proper accounts and records; to use the Government Banking Service.

Governance – for example, to have a governing body and Accountable Officer; to have a published constitution; to publish an annual report; to maintain one or more publicly accessible registers of interest; to make arrangements for managing conflicts of interest.

The same guidance also identifies CCG powers under the same headings. In relation to finance and governance notable powers include the ability to:

- enter into partnership arrangements with local authorities (for example, pooled budgets and lead commissioning)
- enter into contracts to provide services
- act jointly with other CCGs, including pooling commissioning funds for lead/joint commissioning
- make direct payments to patients (subject to regulations)
- pool resources with local authorities
- enter into externally financed development arrangements
- pay governing body members remuneration and travelling or other allowances.

For full details of a CCG's functions, duties and powers refer to the Department of Health guide.

Commissioning support units (CSUs)

Initially all CCGs are obtaining commissioning support services from commissioning support units (CSUs) hosted by NHS England in line with service level agreements (SLAs) that set out what each party to the agreement expects and/or requires. NHS England has set out in guidance 'key minimum clauses' that it would expect to see in these SLAs along with an example agreement and template. After the SLAs expire in October 2014, CCGs can choose where they obtain such services. NHS England is working with CCGs, CSUs and non-NHS providers of support services to develop a strategy that will help CCGs make informed choices in this area. See NHS England's website for more information.

How CCGs are Financed

CCGs receive funding for commissioning NHS services from NHS England. The main allocation is based on a formula that is currently under review to ensure that it supports the aim of improving health outcomes and reducing inequalities. The new formula is expected to be in use for the 2014/15 allocations (see chapter 10 for more details).

CCGs that improve or achieve on four national measures (for example, reducing avoidable emergency admissions and ensuring the roll out of the 'friends and family test') and three local measures set with health and wellbeing boards will also receive a 'quality premium' in the following year (set at £5 per head for each CCG). For details see NHS England's guidance.

There is also a separate running cost allowance which is based on the population served by each CCG's constituent practices adjusted to take account of inaccurate lists and unregistered people. For 2013/14, the allowance is set at a maximum of £25 per head. This allowance must cover all CCG management costs including the costs of commissioning support services. CCGs are free to decide how best to use this allowance to carry out commissioning support activities and may choose to undertake some or all of these roles themselves. They also have the flexibility to use the money to buy in the services needed (for example, data analysis and contract monitoring) from external sources such as a CSU hosted by NHS England. As well as covering the costs directly associated with commissioning, the allowance also covers the costs of the Accountable Officer, Chief Finance Officer, internal and external audit and counter fraud services.

References and Further Reading

Details of the CCG authorisation process, NHS England website:
www.england.nhs.uk/resources/resources-for-ccgs/auth/

Clinical Commissioning Group Governing Body Members: Role Outlines, Attributes and Skills, NHS England, 2012: www.england.nhs.uk/wp-content/uploads/2012/09/ccg-members-roles.pdf

Model Constitution Framework for CCGs, NHS England, 2012:
www.england.nhs.uk/resources/resources-for-ccgs/ccg-mod-cons-framework/

CCG Outcomes Indicator Set, NHS England: www.england.nhs.uk/ccg-ois/

The Functions of Clinical Commissioning Groups, Department of Health, 2012:
www.gov.uk/government/news/functions-of-clinical-commissioning-groups

Information about personal health budgets: www.personalhealthbudgets.england.nhs.uk/

SLAs for CCGs and CSUs – see the CCG resources page of NHS England's website:
www.england.nhs.uk/resources/resources-for-ccgs/

Quality Premium: 2013/14: Guidance for CCGs, NHS England, 2012:
www.england.nhs.uk/wp-content/uploads/2013/03/qual-premium.pdf

Chapter 6: NHS finance – Who Does What?

The Role of Primary Care

> **Overview**
>
> This chapter looks at the main primary care services in the NHS with a focus on what they do and how they are financed. In terms of their position in the NHS structure, primary care services fall within the 'providers' box in the diagram on page 16.

What is Primary Care and Who Provides it?

Primary care is where people normally go when they first develop a health problem – usually this will be a GP but there are many other health professionals in this front line team including nurses, health visitors, dentists, opticians and pharmacists.

In this chapter we are going to focus on providers of primary care services (often referred to as 'primary medical services') and will also look at prescribing (a significant cost to the NHS).

It is worth noting at the outset that, although they are an essential part of the NHS, most family doctors, dentists, opticians and pharmacists are independent contractors or businesses – i.e. they are not NHS employees.

Accountability

Primary care service providers are accountable to:

- the patients to whom they provide services
- NHS England which agrees signed contracts with them for the services provided and outcomes achieved
- the clinical commissioning group (CCG) to which they belong (where that is the case)
- their own professional bodies
- the Care Quality Commission (CQC) for meeting essential standards of quality care.

What Primary Care Providers do

Primary care health providers play a central role in the community. All of us will have some contact with NHS primary care during our lives. General practitioners (GPs) or 'family doctors', pharmacists, dentists and opticians all provide health services to the public. They also act as a gateway to other services. For example, referrals to secondary care in hospitals must come from a primary care practitioner, usually a GP.

How Primary Care is Financed

Primary care services are commissioned by NHS England and financed via contracts that it holds. These contracts are agreed nationally and refreshed each year. Each contract is discussed below.

GP services

At present, there are three main contract types for GP services – General Medical Services (GMS), Personal Medical Services (PMS) and Alternative Provider Medical Services (APMS).

General Medical Services (GMS)

The GMS contract (also known as the GP contract) came into effect in April 2004 and is agreed nationally. This practice-based contract has three main income streams:

GMS Contract – Main Income Streams

A **global sum** to cover running costs and the provision of 'essential' and 'additional' services – this is calculated through a resource allocation formula based on the age/sex of the practice's population, additional needs, list turnover, nursing home patients and rurality. In addition to general running costs, this global sum covers the provision of essential and additional services. Essential services, which have to be provided by every practice, cover the care of patients during an episode of illness, the general management of chronic disease and care for the terminally ill. Additional services, such as contraceptive services, child health surveillance and out of hours services are voluntary. Practices that opt out of providing additional services have their global sum reduced by a nationally agreed percentage rate.

The **Quality and Outcomes Framework** (QOF) to reward improved standards in both clinical and non-clinical areas – this sets out a range of standards across four headings: clinical; public health; quality and productivity and patient experience. Practices are awarded points for achieving these standards, set out in a range of indicators, and receive a set payment per point. Although participation in QOF is voluntary, most GP practices take part.

Enhanced service payments – to meet the costs of extra specialised services or essential services that are delivered to a higher standard. There are two types of enhanced services:

* Directed Enhanced Services (DES) that **must** be commissioned (for example, childhood immunisation and alcohol reduction)
* Local Enhanced Services (LES) that are optional and are commissioned by local negotiation to meet specific local needs (for example, enhanced medical care for asylum seekers or non-English speakers).

Since April 2013, NHS England has been responsible for commissioning enhanced services nationally (equivalent to DES) although it may devolve responsibility for managing some of them to CCGs. Although NHS England retains the ability to commission LES, it is unlikely to do so. Instead, CCGs are expected to decide how best to use local resources to invest in community based services that are beyond the scope of the GP contract.

There are also funding streams for GP practices to cover:

- **premises**: under the terms of the GMS contract, practices are reimbursed for their premises costs. This includes rent and rates charges incurred. A notional rent payment is made to practices that own their premises
- **seniority pay**: this is paid at nationally agreed rates and is dependent upon the number of years a GP has worked in the NHS
- **locum cover**: practices may receive a contribution towards the costs of employing a locum to cover maternity, paternity and sickness of a partner
- **information communications and technology (ICT)**: responsibility for the delivery of primary care information services rests with NHS England. However, it has delegated responsibility (and the associated funding) for the operational management of GP IT services to CCGs. CCGs can commission these services from any provider that meets a set of quality standards that have been set by NHS England in conjunction with CCGs.

The GMS contract tends to be adjusted annually with the payment provisions set out in detail in the 'Statement of Financial Entitlements (SFE)'. At present around 53% of practices have GMS contracts.

Personal Medical Services (PMS)

PMS contracts were introduced in 1998 and allow the provider GP to negotiate a local agreement with their commissioners in line with local healthcare needs. This means that GPs are paid contract sums to deliver a defined service. PMS practices are also able to receive quality payments and are eligible for enhanced services payments (if these are not already in their PMS contract) plus the premises, ICT and seniority pay. Currently around 44% of practices receive their funding under locally agreed PMS contracts. PMS practices can opt to switch into the GMS contract.

Alternative Provider Medical Services (APMS)

APMS contracts are provided under directions of the Secretary of State for Health and can be let to private sector, voluntary and not-for-profit providers of general medical services as well as to traditional GP practices, NHS and foundation trusts. APMS contracts tend to be used in areas of historic under provision or to 're-provide' services where GP practices have opted out. They can also be used to improve access where GP recruitment and retention is a problem. Currently around 3% of GP services are delivered under APMS contracts.

Out of hours services

Since April 2004, GP practices have been able to opt out of providing out of hours services and around 90% of GMS and PMS practices have gone down this route. From April 2013, CCGs are responsible for commissioning out of hours services for those practices that have opted out. Where out of hours services are still provided by GP practices under the GMS/PMS contract (i.e. the 10% who did not opt out), NHS England is responsible for their commissioning as in such instances, they remain an integral part of the GMS/PMS contract.

Dental services

Most primary dental care (i.e. the main dental care needed to maintain good oral health) is provided by self-employed dentists or corporate bodies that hold contracts with the NHS. At present there are two types of contract.

Dental Contracts

General Dental Services (GDS) – this contract came into force in 2006 and pays dentists a set value for an agreed number of units of dental activity (UDAs). A reform of patients' charges came into effect at the same time with the introduction of three bands depending on the type of treatment received.

Personal Dental Services (PDS) – under this contract, practices are paid a set contract value in return for having an agreed number of patients on their list. The contract is designed to give a 10% decrease in working time to allow dentists to use 5% to give access slots to unregistered patients to be seen urgently, and 5% to take them off the 'treadmill' of items of service payments.

Both GDS and PDS contracts are negotiated locally using national regulations. The key difference is that PDS contracts are time limited and GDS contracts are not.

As with GP contracts, payments for GDS and PDS contracts are made in line with a SFE that covers reimbursements for services provided and payments related to dentists' employment. All dentists under both GDS and PDS contracts must provide a full range of general dental services plus any agreed additional services.

The Government plans to introduce a new national dental contract based on registration, capitation and quality. This will mean that dentists will be paid on a 'per patient' rather than a 'per treatment' basis and rewarded for continuity and quality of care. A number of different contract models were piloted at 70 sites throughout England up until March 2013 with another 25 pilot sites now 'fine tuning' different parts of the new contract. Subject to the results of the pilots and parliamentary approval, the intention is that the new contract will be introduced from April 2014.

Since April 2013, NHS England has been responsible for commissioning all NHS dental services as part of its direct commissioning responsibilities. This includes primary dental care, dental hospitals and out of hours services.

Pharmacy services

In April 2005, a 'new' community pharmacy contract came into effect which has since been re-negotiated annually. This contract specifies three levels of service.

Pharmacy Services – the three Levels of Service

1. Essential services – services that **must** be provided by all pharmacies. For example, dispensing and repeat dispensing; disposal of unwanted medicines; promoting healthy lifestyles; signposting and support for self-care
2. Advanced services – services that **may** be provided by accredited pharmacists and pharmacies. For example, medicine use reviews (MURs) and the new medicine service (NMS)
3. Enhanced services – services that may be commissioned to meet local needs, including stop smoking schemes, emergency hormonal contraception and minor ailments.

From April 2013, NHS England is responsible for commissioning community pharmacy services as part of its direct commissioning activities. CCGs and local authorities can also commission some services that are not covered by the pharmacy contract directly from community pharmacists – where they do this they must agree the specification and payment terms locally.

In relation to the supply and dispensing of drugs, NHS Prescriptions Services (part of the NHS Business Services Authority) receives details of all prescriptions dispensed in England, and then calculates the amounts payable, allowing for the drug and container cost and a service fee.

An electronic prescription service (EPS) is also being developed – this allows prescribers (such as GPs and practice nurses) to send prescriptions electronically to a dispenser of the patient's choice, thus making the prescribing and dispensing process safer and more convenient. Community pharmacies receive payments for signing up to the scheme and updating their systems. They also receive monthly payments for using the system.

Ophthalmic services

The basis on which payments are made for optical services is set out in the *NHS Act 2006* which introduced three tiers of service.

> **Ophthalmic Services – the three Tiers of Service**
>
> 1. Mandatory (or 'essential') – services that all commissioners **must** commission and which any eligible contractor can provide: i.e. the provision of NHS sight tests
> 2. Additional – services that all commissioners must commission but not all contractors are obliged to provide. For example, the provision of sight tests in alternative settings such as a nursing home
> 3. Enhanced – services that a commissioner may choose to commission and fund to meet local needs.

Payments for NHS sight tests for 'eligible patients' (i.e. patients who meet set criteria – for example, children under 16 and adults over 60) are made in accordance with the Department of Health's 'general ophthalmic services' (GOS) regulations. Only fees for eligible patients are met from the NHS budget – all other patients pay privately for these services.

From April 2013 NHS England must commission mandatory and additional services as part of its direct commissioning function and is able to commission enhanced services. CCGs can also commission enhanced services directly from providers on a locally agreed basis (i.e. they are outside the GOS contract).

Prescribing

The rising cost of primary care prescribing (over £8 billion each year) is a significant cost pressure with drug inflation regularly outstripping inflation on other budgets. Prescribing costs have always risen faster than general inflation as new, more effective and more expensive drugs become available. However, this has become even more pronounced in recent years partly as a result of guidance from the National Institute for Health and Care Excellence (NICE).

One of NICE's roles is to assess the clinical and cost-effectiveness of new drugs and technologies and this has an impact on both prescription volume and cost. The effects are mitigated to an extent by securing efficiencies from improvements in prescribing practice.

From a financing viewpoint, prescribing is not covered in GPs or dentists contracts. Instead, as mentioned earlier, the costs of drugs prescribed are calculated by NHS Prescription Services and charged to the relevant CCG (for GP prescriptions) and to NHS England (for dentists). The associated dispensing fees are met by NHS England.

References and Further Reading

NHS primary care commissioning information – NHS England:
www.england.nhs.uk/resources/resource-primary/

GMS contract information:
www.nhsemployers.org/PayAndContracts/GeneralMedicalServicesContract/Pages/Contract.aspx

Quality and Outcomes Framework: www.nhsemployers.org/PayAndContracts/
GeneralMedicalServicesContract/QOF/Pages/QualityOutcomesFramework.aspx

Enhanced Services Commissioning Fact Sheet, NHS England, 2012:
www.england.nhs.uk/wp-content/uploads/2012/03/fact-enhanced-serv.pdf

GP IT Services: Operating Model, NHS England, 2012: www.england.nhs.uk/2012/12/04/gp-it/

Statement of Financial Entitlements (archived web pages):
http://webarchive.nationalarchives.gov.uk/+/www.dh.gov.uk/en/Healthcare/Primarycare/PMC/
contractingroutes/DH_4133079

Dental contract pilots information and background:
www.gov.uk/government/publications/extension-to-dental-contract-pilot-scheme

For information about general ophthalmic services regulations and contracts the Local Optical Committee Support Unit's website is helpful: www.locsu.co.uk/regulation/

Pharmacy contract information:
www.nhsemployers.org/PayAndContracts/CommunityPharmacyContract/
CPCFservicedevelopments2011/Pages/CPCF-service-developments-2011_12.aspx

NHS Prescription Services: www.nhsbsa.nhs.uk/prescriptionservices.aspx

Information on prescribing and the Electronic Prescription Service, Health and Social Care Information Centre: www.hscic.gov.uk/prescribing

Chapter 7: NHS finance – Who Does What?

The Role of Community, Secondary and Tertiary Care Providers

> **Overview**
>
> This chapter looks at the main providers of community, secondary and tertiary care in the NHS with a focus on their roles, responsibilities, financing and governance. To remind yourself of where providers sit in the NHS structure, look back at the diagram on page 16.

What is Community Care?

Community care – as its name suggests – is the term used for those health services provided in community settings such as patients' homes, GP practices and (small) community hospitals.

> **Community Care Services – Examples**
>
> * Community health services
> * Mental health services
> * Support for people with learning disabilities
> * Services for physically disabled people
> * Community-based care for elderly people (for example, community hospitals)
> * Virtual wards
> * Telehealth, telecare and telemedicine

What is Secondary Care?

Secondary care is healthcare usually provided in a hospital setting (for example, a 'district general' or acute hospital) following a referral from a primary care professional.

What is Tertiary Care?

Tertiary care comprises those services provided in a limited number of specialist units usually in the larger or teaching hospitals – for example, cardiac surgery or neurology. Often these services are accessed by a referral from one consultant to another. However, in larger hospitals that provide tertiary care services themselves, referral can take place directly on admission.

Who Provides Community, Secondary and Tertiary Services?

Community, secondary and tertiary services can be commissioned from 'any qualified provider (AQP)' – in other words, any provider that is registered with the Care Quality Commission (CQC) and licenced by Monitor. Examples of AQPs include NHS organisations, private sector healthcare providers (for example, Virgin Health), voluntary or charitable sector providers and social enterprise organisations.

This chapter's primary focus is on NHS organisations and in particular community, mental health, acute, ambulance and foundation trusts across England. However, we will also look briefly at the part played by social enterprise organisations.

Community, Mental Health, Ambulance and Acute (non-foundation) NHS trusts

What they are – constitution, structure and accountabilities

Constitution

NHS trusts were formed from 1991 onwards under the *NHS and Community Care Act 1990*. All NHS hospitals in England providing acute and mental health services are part of an NHS trust and in some areas they also host community services. NHS trusts provide mainly, but not exclusively, hospital-based secondary care services. The most common type is an acute hospital trust but there are also mental health, community and ambulance trusts. Some trusts act as regional or national centres of expertise for more specialised care, while others are attached to universities and help to train health professionals.

Over recent years there has been growth in the number of community NHS trusts. Often these have been formed as stand-alone organisations from the former 'provider arms' of primary care trusts (PCTs) but other NHS trusts can also host or provide community services.

Structure

All NHS trusts (including community trusts) have a Board whose make up is set out in primary legislation under *The NHS Trusts (Membership and Procedure) Regulations 1990*.

Each NHS or community trust Board has a maximum number of twelve directors excluding the Chair; up to seven non-executive members (although the majority have five) and no more than five executive directors. For mental health trusts, the Board size is a maximum of 14 (excluding the Chair) which includes no more than seven non-executive directors (NEDs) and seven executive directors. Since April 2013, the NHS Trust Development Authority (NHS TDA) has been responsible for appointing NEDs.

Within the Board's executive directors, each trust must have:

- a Chief Officer (the Chief Executive who is also the 'Accountable Officer' – see below)
- a Chief Finance Officer (the Finance Director)
- a medical or dental practitioner and registered nurse or midwife (except in the case of ambulance trusts).

Other executive directors may attend Board meetings (in addition to the Chief Executive and Chief Finance Officer) but do not hold the full range of responsibilities – for example, they do not have the right to vote on Board decisions. Also, although the medical and nursing professions must be represented at Board level, this can be via the Chief Executive if she or he has a medical or nursing background.

An NHS trust Board is collectively responsible for promoting the success of the organisation by directing and supervising its affairs. This involves:

- setting the organisation's values and standards and ensuring that its obligations to patients, the local community and the Secretary of State are understood and met
- providing active leadership of the organisation within a framework of prudent and effective controls that enable risk to be assessed and managed
- setting the organisation's strategic aims
- ensuring that the necessary financial and human resources are in place for the organisation to meet its objectives
- reviewing management performance.

All remaining (non-foundation) NHS trusts are expected to achieve foundation status as swiftly as they can but there is no longer a 'blanket deadline'. To help them work towards this goal, trusts are monitored and supported by the NHS TDA (see chapter 3). Once all trusts have achieved foundation status the legislation that allows their establishment will be repealed.

Accountabilities

In terms of accountability, an NHS trust's Chief Executive is the 'Accountable Officer'. This is a statutory role and means that he or she is accountable to the Department of Health's Accounting Officer (via the NHS TDA's Accounting Officer) and ultimately to Parliament (see chapter 13 for more about the role of the Accountable Officer). As well as this formal accountability line, trusts are accountable to their patients and to the commissioners of their services (via contracts). In addition there is a system of independent inspection and regulation by external organisations such as the Care Quality Commission (see chapter 9).

What they do – roles and responsibilities

All NHS trusts are required to have regard to the *NHS Constitution*, provide high-quality healthcare and spend their money efficiently. They must also decide how the services they deliver will develop and improve.

> The NHS Constitution sets out the:
>
> - **Rights** to which patients, public and staff are entitled
> - **Pledges** which the NHS is committed to achieve
> - **Responsibilities** that the public, patients and staff owe to one another

Community NHS trusts specialise in delivering NHS care in patients' homes and in community settings – for example in nursing homes, clinics, community hospitals, minor injury units, walk-in centres and mobile units. These trusts employ a range of staff including community and district nurses, physiotherapists, school nurses, health visitors, rehabilitation and palliative care specialists and dieticians.

Acute NHS trusts run hospitals and employ clinical staff (for example, nurses, doctors, pharmacists, and midwives); related therapeutic specialists (for example, physiotherapists, radiographers, podiatrists, speech and language therapists, counsellors, occupational therapists and psychologists) and non-clinical staff (for example, porters, cleaners, managers, engineers, caterers and domestic and security staff).

Mental health NHS trusts provide health and social care services for people with mental health problems or learning disabilities.

Ambulance trusts provide emergency access to healthcare and patient transport services.

To find out more about each type of trust visit the NHS Choices website.

How they are financed

Revenue financing

NHS trusts receive revenue income (to meet the costs of their day-today running) from a number of sources including those set out below:

Revenue Income Sources

Through the commissioning process with NHS England, clinical commissioning groups (CCGs) and other NHS trusts – this usually represents 75% to 90% of total income. Trusts are commissioned to provide services for patients and are paid in line with a standard NHS contract agreed before the start of each financial year.

Specific funding to those trusts providing nursing, medical and non-medical staff education and training services (generally based on numbers in training).

Allocations where trusts are undertaking agreed research and development.

Charges made for 'hosted services' (for example, internal audit consortia).

Charges to staff, visitors or patients for services provided, such as catering, car parking or the provision of private patient facilities.

Grants from other government bodies or charitable organisations.

The NHS injury cost recovery scheme – this allows the NHS to reclaim the cost of treating injured patients in all cases where personal injury compensation is paid.

The levels of income received from these various sources will vary between different types of NHS trust – for example, community trusts are unlikely to have income generation schemes or injury costs income (unless they run minor injury units).

In addition, a very limited number of NHS trusts have Ministry of Defence (MOD) hospital units. Where this is the case, the trust will have two contracts: one for training military medical personnel and one for treating military patients. Income relating to the treatment contract is paid directly to the trust by the MOD. The contract for treating military personnel mirrors the

NHS standard contract and uses payment by results (see chapter 18) although it may contain the opportunity for additional 'premia' payments for treating military personnel more quickly.

Capital financing

NHS trusts have two main sources of capital funding (to fund the purchase of new and replacement assets such as buildings and equipment):

- internally generated funds (via retained surpluses, depreciation and proceeds from the sale of capital assets)
- capital investment loans from the Department of Health.

Access to capital funding is linked to financial performance and affordability with a 'borrowing limit' (sometimes referred to as a 'prudential borrowing limit' or PBL) set for each trust. This limit indicates the maximum cumulative borrowing that a trust may take on to fund additional capital investment and to finance operations generally.

NHS trusts may also have access to other forms of capital financing including:

- charitable donations
- a private finance initiative (PFI) contract with the private sector
- local improvement finance trust (LIFT) funding for community projects.

If you would like to find out more about capital funding (including borrowing limits), see chapter 15.

NHS Foundation Trusts

What they are – constitution, structure and accountabilities

Constitution

NHS foundation trusts (FTs) were created as new legal entities in the form of public benefit corporations by the *Health and Social Care (Community Health and Standards) Act 2003* – now consolidated in the *NHS Act 2006*. This model draws on the traditions of mutual organisations established under the Industrial and Provident legislation. In practice this means that every FT has a duty to consult and involve a Council of Governors (comprising staff, patients, members of the public and other key stakeholders) in strategic planning.

The first FTs appeared in 2004 and since then the numbers have steadily grown. The Government expects all remaining NHS trusts to achieve foundation status (or be integrated into an existing foundation trust) as swiftly as possible but there is no longer a 'blanket deadline'.

The FT structure represents a model of local management where central government involvement is reduced. However, it is important to remember that FTs remain part of the NHS with the primary purpose of providing NHS services to NHS patients according to NHS principles and standards.

The most significant distinguishing feature of FTs is that they are not directly accountable to the Department of Health. Instead their functions are managed and executed through a Council of Governors and a Board of Directors and they are regulated by Monitor (see chapter 9 for more about Monitor and its regulatory regime).

The Council of Governors

Governors of FTs are representative of the local community and provide a link between the trusts and its patients, service users and stakeholders. These governors consist of both elected and appointed individuals drawn from FT members and other stakeholder groups (including the public, patients and staff). When applying to be a member of an FT, an individual applicant can also confirm an interest in becoming a governor. The Council of Governors is required to hold the FT to account.

The Board of Directors

Every FT must have an effective Board of Directors that consists of executive directors (which must include the Chief Executive and Chief Finance Officer) and NEDs. The Chair of the Board must be a NED. NEDs should have particular experience or skills that help the Board function well. They are appointed by the Council of Governors based on recommendations made by a 'nominations committee'.

The Board of Directors is collectively responsible for every decision it takes regardless of individual directors' skills or status. In particular, the Board of Directors must set the FT's strategic aims (taking account of the views of the Council of Governors) and is responsible for 'ensuring compliance by the NHS foundation trust with its terms of authorisation [now its licence], its constitution, mandatory guidance issued by Monitor, relevant statutory requirements and contractual obligations'.[1] Meetings of the Board of Directors must be open to the public.

The Accounting Officer

The FT's Chief Executive is also the 'Accounting Officer' (a role known as the 'Accountable Officer' in most other NHS organisations). This is a statutory role originally set out in the 2003 Act which provides the formal accountability link from the FT to parliament. The Accounting Officer's duties are set out in a memorandum issued by Monitor that states that 'Accounting Officers are responsible to parliament for the resources under their control'.

As well as the formal accountability line from the Accounting Officer, FTs (like other trusts) are accountable to both their patients and to the commissioners of their services (via contracts). In addition there is a system of independent inspection and regulation by organisations such as the Care Quality Commission (see chapter 9).

---

[1] *Code of Governance for NHS Foundation Trusts*, Monitor, 2010.

What FTs do – roles and responsibilities

Although FTs are independent they remain part of the NHS with the primary purpose of providing NHS services to NHS patients according to NHS principles and standards. In particular, the public continues to receive healthcare according to core NHS principles – free care, based on need and not the ability to pay.

As with non-foundation NHS trusts, there are FTs that provide acute, tertiary, mental health, community and ambulance services across England.

How FTs are financed

Revenue financing

FTs (like non-foundation trusts) receive revenue income (to meet the costs of their day-to-day running) from a number of sources including:

- through the commissioning process with NHS England, CCGs and other NHS trusts – this usually represents 75% to 90% of total income. FTs are commissioned to provide services for patients and are paid in line with a standard NHS contract agreed before the start of each financial year
- specific funding to those FTs providing nursing, medical and non-medical staff education and training services (generally based on numbers in training)
- allocations where FTs are undertaking agreed research and development
- charges made for 'hosted services' (for example, internal audit consortia)
- charges to staff, visitors or patients for services provided, such as catering, car parking or the provision of private patient facilities
- grants from other government bodies or charitable organisations
- the NHS injury cost recovery scheme – this allows the NHS to reclaim the cost of treating injured patients in all cases where personal injury compensation is paid.

As with other non-foundation trusts, a very small number of FTs have a Ministry of Defence (MOD) hospital unit within their trust. Where this is the case, the FT will have two contracts: one for training military medical personnel and one for treating military patients. Income relating to the treatment contract is paid directly to the FT by the MOD. The contract for treating military personnel mirrors the standard NHS contract and uses payment by results (see chapter 18) although it may contain the opportunity for additional 'premia' payments for treating military personnel more quickly.

Income from private patients

Many FTs generate additional income through treating patients privately: either billing insurance companies or individuals direct. Until 1st October 2012, FTs were restricted in the amount of income they could generate in this way by the 'private patient income cap'. However, this cap has now been removed and instead FTs must 'ensure that their total income from NHS-funded goods and services is greater than their total income from any other sources'. They must also produce separate accounts for NHS and private-funded services.

Other commercial ventures

Many FTs are developing other commercial sources of income at home and abroad. For example, Moorfields Eye Hospital NHS Foundation Trust has operated an eye hospital in Dubai since 2006 which contributed a surplus of £0.3 million in 2011/12. In addition, a new scheme announced in August 2012 by the Department of Health and the UK Trade and Investment Department will enable NHS organisations to sell their services abroad on a larger scale.

Interest and investment income

FTs are allowed to retain surplus cash balances which can be invested and generate a return for the organisation. Each FT is required to have a policy for these investments that is approved by its Board.

Capital financing

Prior to the *Health and Social Care Act 2012*, capital financing for FTs was governed by Monitor's *Prudential Borrowing Code*. This involved Monitor setting a limit each year on borrowing for each FT that determined how readily capital and working capital could be accessed and the maximum cumulative amount that an FT could borrow.

The Code no longer applies. Instead, the 2012 Act established new requirements for the Department of Health to produce guidance in relation to the powers that it has to lend to FTs – see chapter 15.

As with non-foundation NHS trusts, the main source of capital funding is from internally generated resources (i.e. retained surpluses, depreciation and proceeds from the sale of capital assets). For larger schemes an FT has to date been able to borrow from the Foundation Trust Financing Facility (FTFF) as well as from the open market, including commercial loans from banks and other private lending organisations. However, as all borrowing must be repaid, an FT must always consider affordability.

Other possible sources of funding for capital projects include:

* working in partnership with the private sector – most commonly using the private finance initiative (PFI)
* charitable donations.

See chapter 15 for more details about capital funding and planning.

Social Enterprise Organisations (SEOs)

What they are – constitution, structure and accountabilities

A social enterprise organisation is a business that has mainly social aims with any surpluses re-invested in its services or the community. There is a wide variety of SEOs in the UK, ranging from community-owned village shops to large organisations such as the Eden Project. SEOs differ from charity or voluntary sector organisations as they generate the majority of their income through the trading of goods or services rather than via donations.

In terms of regulation and accountability, SEOs are not part of the NHS – instead they are stand-alone not-for-profit businesses. Any SEO that wishes to provide services to NHS patients must therefore be registered with the CQC and (in future) licenced by Monitor.

There is a range of SEO models operating in health and social care including mutual, co-operative or employee owned organisations and community interest companies (CICs). Many are single service providers (for example, speech and language therapy or podiatry) but there are around 40 that were set up as a result of the 'transforming community services (TCS)' programme which removed provider activities from primary care trusts. These tend to provide a full range of community services including district nursing, health visiting and school nursing.

Examples of SEOs

Central Surrey Health is co-owned by its employees and provides community nursing and therapy services.

In the South West there are five social enterprises that were formed in October 2011 as a result of the TCS agenda. In this case, each organisation was established as a CIC – a type of social enterprise set up specifically for organisations operating for the benefit of the community rather than for the benefit of shareholders.

For an SEO to be constituted as a CIC, it must pass a 'community interest test' that shows the company will benefit the community it was set up to serve. There is also an 'asset lock' which means that any surpluses made must be reinvested for the good of the community. CICs are granted their status by the CIC Regulator and registered with Companies House. CIC accounts are submitted in line with Companies House timetables rather than those of the NHS.

For more information visit the CIC regulator's website: www.cicregulator.gov.uk

What SEOs do

SEOs are commissioned to provide services to NHS patients to meet local needs.

How SEOs are financed

For SEOs established under TCS, the bulk of their funding is derived from the same NHS route as if they had been set up as a Community NHS Trust. In such cases, budgets from the PCT provider arm were often rolled over into block contracts, usually to cover a set period of time (of say 4 years) before being re-tendered. However, there are opportunities for SEOs to expand the range of services they deliver and hence the number of commissioners served and income received – for example, by providing services previously delivered by local authorities or forming subsidiary companies (such as 'charitable arms') to take advantage of tax opportunities and enable the receipt of charitable donations.

References and Further Reading

Information about the 'Any Qualified Provider' approach:
https://www.supply2health.nhs.uk/AQPResourceCentre/Pages/AQPHome.aspx

NHS and Community Care Act 1990: www.legislation.gov.uk/ukpga/1990/19/contents

The NHS Trusts (Membership and Procedure) Regulations 1990:
www.legislation.gov.uk/uksi/1990/2024/contents/made

NHS Trust Development Authority: www.ntda.nhs.uk/

The NHS Constitution for England, Department of Health, 2013:
www.gov.uk/government/publications/the-nhs-constitution-for-england

Information about types of NHS trust – NHS Choices website:
www.nhs.uk/NHSEngland/thenhs/about/Pages/authoritiesandtrusts.aspx

NHS standard contract information: www.england.nhs.uk/nhs-standard-contract/

NHS Act 2006: www.legislation.gov.uk/ukpga/2006/41/contents

Code of Governance for NHS Foundation Trusts, Monitor, 2010:
www.monitor-nhsft.gov.uk/home/news-events-and-publications/our-publications/browse-category/guidance-foundation-trusts/mandat-3

Information about FTs and private patient income: www.monitor-nhsft.gov.uk/home/news-events-and-publications/latest-press-releases/monitor-update-private-patient-income-cap-nh

Information about transforming community services:
http://healthandcare.dh.gov.uk/category/nhs-providers/tcs/

For more about community interest companies: www.bis.gov.uk/cicregulator/

Chapter 8: NHS Finance – Who Does What?

The Role of Local Authorities, Health and Wellbeing Boards and HealthWatch

> Overview
>
> This chapter looks at the role of local authorities with a focus on how they work with (and link to) the NHS. In particular, it looks at the practical implications of the new duties placed on local authorities as a result of the *Health and Social Care Act 2012* and at the ways in which local authorities and the NHS work together. To see where they fit into the NHS structure, refer to the diagram on page 16.

Local Authorities – what are they?

Local authorities provide public services to local communities and are run by democratically elected councillors who are accountable to their electorate. In England, there is a mixture of single tier and two tier local authority areas. Where there are two tiers of local government, the upper tier is usually known as the county council and the lower tier as the district, borough or city council. Unitary authorities (i.e. where there is a single tier) can go by any of these names.

How Local Authorities Link to the NHS

NHS organisations have long been expected to engage with their local communities to improve health and wellbeing and reduce health inequalities. For many years, this has involved NHS organisations working in partnership with local authorities to manage and deliver services in which both parties have an interest. In addition, although the Department of Health is responsible for setting national policy for adult social care and securing its funding from the Treasury within the spending review process (see chapter 10), local authorities deliver the services.

As a result of the 2012 Act, the role of local authorities has been strengthened to help fulfil the Coalition Government's objective that, through the involvement of elected councillors, local authorities will bring greater local democratic legitimacy to the NHS and have more influence over commissioning, particularly in relation to public health and social care. The Act is also designed to make it easier to 'further integrate health with adult social care, children's services (including education) and wider services, including disability services, housing, and tackling crime and disorder.'

As a result, local authorities now have a statutory responsibility to join up commissioning of NHS services, social care, public health and health improvement. They are also required to:

- jointly appoint a Director of Public Health in conjunction with Public Health England
- jointly commission some services with clinical commissioning groups (CCGs)
- lead joint strategic needs assessments (JSNAs) and joint health and wellbeing strategies

(JHWS) to ensure coherent and co-coordinated commissioning strategies (a role carried out jointly with CCGs via health and wellbeing boards – see below)

* support local voice, and the exercise of patient choice
* lead on local health improvement and prevention activity.

In practice, this means that much of the joint working that has gone on for years will continue but local authorities now have additional statutory responsibilities in relation to health improvement and receive a ring fenced grant from the NHS allocation.

Local Authorities' Statutory Roles and Responsibilities in Relation to the NHS

Health and wellbeing boards

To reflect local authorities' strengthened role, every upper tier local authority must establish a 'health and wellbeing board' (HWB) to provide a forum for public accountability and join up commissioning across the NHS, social care, public health and other services relating to health and wellbeing. Core membership of each HWB must include members of CCGs, the Director of Adult Social Services, the Director of Children's Services, the Director of Public Health, local HealthWatch (see later on in this chapter) and at least one democratically elected councillor. HWBs can also require the attendance of NHS England when relevant.

HWBs were established in shadow form in 2012/13 and assumed their powers and duties as statutory committees of local authorities in April 2013. As mentioned above, their remit is to lead the development of the JSNA and the new high level JHWS (see below). They also have a duty to involve service users and the public and work with CCGs to ensure that commissioning plans meet local needs. This approach is designed to provide strategic co-ordination to the commissioning of NHS services, social care and health improvement.

HWBs are financed by local authorities and are accountable to communities, service users and local authority overview and scrutiny committees. Individual representatives on HWBs are also accountable for the decisions taken to their own organisations and as a result, HWBs are accountable to individual member organisations.

Joint strategic needs assessments

JSNAs are designed to 'identify the current and future health and wellbeing needs of a local population'[1] and have been in place since their introduction in section 116 of *the Local Government and Public Involvement in Health Act 2007*. The *Health and Social Care Act 2012* retains JSNAs but places the responsibility for producing them jointly on local authorities and CCGs. The Act also requires local authorities and CCGs to undertake the JSNA through the HWB so in practice, it is the HWB that pulls the strategy together with local authorities and CCGs ultimately responsible for them and required to 'have regard to them' when exercising their functions.

---

[1] *Guidance on Joint Strategic Needs Assessment*, Departments of Health and Communities and Local Government, 2007.

Joint health and wellbeing strategies

In addition, the 2012 Act requires local authorities and CCGs to produce (again via the HWB) a joint health and wellbeing strategy (JHWS) that sets out plans to address the needs of the local population and reduce inequalities identified in the JSNA. NHS and local authority commissioners must then 'have regard to' the JHWS when exercising their functions.

Health improvement

As mentioned above, the 2012 Act introduces a new statutory duty on affected local authorities (upper tier and unitary) to improve the health of the local population. The Act also gives the Secretary of State the power to require local authorities to carry out certain health protection functions and to prescribe how they carry out their health improvement activities. There are also new statutory arrangements for local authority leadership in this area, complemented by the creation of Public Health England (PHE) – with local Directors of Public Health being appointed jointly by local authorities and PHE. These local directors have a ring-fenced health improvement grant to deliver national and local priorities (the grant is allocated by PHE). There is direct accountability to both the local authority, and (through PHE) to the Secretary of State. As they are employed by the local authority, local Directors of Public Health advise councillors and are part of the senior management team of the local authority.

At a practical level, local authorities are responsible for commissioning a range of health improvement services. A limited number of these services are mandated by Government via regulations under section 6c of the *NHS Act 2006*. Other services can be commissioned on a discretionary basis guided by the *Public Health Outcomes Framework*, the JSNA and the JHWS.

Mandatory Services – Examples

- To deliver the NHS Health Check
- To provide population based public health advice to NHS commissioners
- To provide comprehensive sexual health services (excluding abortion, contraceptive services and HIV treatment)

Discretionary Services – Examples

- Lifestyle interventions (for example, to promote physical activity, improve diet and prevent obesity)
- Drug and alcohol misuse services
- Stop smoking services
- Local initiatives to reduce seasonal mortality

As well as commissioning services themselves, local authorities can also work with CCGs and NHS England to make sure services are integrated.

As with other local services, local authorities are accountable primarily to their electorates for work on improving health.

As far as the NHS money is concerned, there are additional accountability mechanisms – specifically:

- PHE publishes data about national and local performance against the *Public Health Outcomes Framework* so local people can see how their local authority is doing
- each local authority Chief Finance Officer must provide a 'statement of grant' showing how the allocation has been spent
- each Director of Public Health must produce (and each local authority publish) an annual report.

Although the Department of Health can incentivise progress in health improvement via the use of a 'health premium', it does not performance manage local authorities or set targets for them.

Local HealthWatch

Local HealthWatch developed from Local Involvement Networks (LINks) with a representative membership of different healthcare users, one of whom sits on the HWB. HealthWatch services are contracted by local authorities with the aim of promoting patient and public involvement and seeking views on local health and social care services.

Local HealthWatch powers are wider than those of LINks as they are designed to be 'more like a 'citizen's advice bureau' for health and social care'. At the national level there is 'HealthWatch England' (described as a 'powerful new consumer champion') which is established as a committee of the Care Quality Commission. The Chair of HealthWatch England is appointed by the Secretary of State and has a seat on the CQC's Board.

Although CCGs are not accountable formally to their local HealthWatch, they have to think about how best to interact with this service.

Local HealthWatch organisations are financed via contracts with the relevant local authorities and are accountable to them for their ability to operate effectively and provide value for money.

Local strategic partnerships

Section 82 of the *NHS Act 2006* requires NHS bodies and local authorities to co-operate with each other 'to secure and advance the health and welfare of the people of England and Wales'. In England local strategic partnerships (LSPs) have been used to help achieve this aim. Where they are in place, LSPs operate at a strategic level and are led by local authorities. LSPs are non-statutory, non-executive, multi-agency bodies that are designed to bring together at local level different parts of the public sector (including the NHS) as well as the private and voluntary sectors so that initiatives and services can support each other and work together.

Overview and scrutiny

Since January 2003, local authorities with social services responsibilities have been able to establish committees of councillors to provide overview and scrutiny of local NHS bodies by virtue of powers set out in section 38 of the *Local Government Act 2000*. The aim is to secure health improvement for local communities by encouraging authorities to look beyond their own service responsibilities to issues of wider concern to local people. This is achieved by giving democratically elected representatives the right to scrutinise how local health services are provided and developed for their constituents. Health organisations are often invited to attend formal meetings of local authorities to answer questions on key issues or to undertake formal consultation with elected members.

The 2012 Act extends the scrutiny role of local authorities to cover any provider of NHS funded services. It also gives local authorities the ability to discharge their health scrutiny functions in 'the way they deem most suitable', taking account of the role of local HealthWatch.

Delayed discharges

Delayed discharges from hospitals (often referred to as 'bed blocking') remains a problem for the NHS and the Government is keen to see the NHS, local authorities and other local organisations (including housing organisations, primary care and the independent and voluntary sectors) working together to minimise the impact. To encourage local authorities to do all they can to make swift discharges possible, a system was introduced by *the Community Care (Delayed Discharges etc) Act 2003* that requires the relevant local authority to reimburse the trust concerned if a patient is delayed from being discharged solely because a community care package is not in place. As part of this arrangement, trusts must notify social services departments of patients who may require community care.

In addition, if a patient is deemed to be medically ready for discharge and delayed discharge payments have been imposed on local authorities under the 2003 Act, commissioners are not liable for any further long stay payments under payment by results (see chapter 18 for more on PbR).

Care trusts

Until April 2013, there were 11 formal care trusts operating across England. These trusts were statutory NHS bodies to which local authorities could delegate health-related functions with the aim of providing integrated health and social care to the local community. Care trusts were established on a voluntary partnership basis where there was joint agreement at local level that this model offered the best way of delivering improved health and social care services. The idea was that by combining NHS and local authority health responsibilities under a single management, continuity of care was improved and administration simplified. Local authority services were delegated to care trusts, not transferred.

In April 2013, care trusts ceased to exist with NHS England's area teams assuming their responsibilities.

Other Approaches to Partnership Working between Local Authorities and the NHS

Section 75 flexibilities

There are a number of arrangements for joint working between NHS organisations and local authorities that were first introduced under section 31 of the *Health Act 1999* – now section 75 of the *NHS Act 2006*. These so-called 'section 75 flexibilities' include:

- pooled budgets
- aligned budgets
- lead commissioning
- integrated provision.

The 2012 Act allows all these section 75 flexibilities to continue but places a duty on CCGs and local authorities (through the HWB) to consider how to make best use of the flexibilities when drawing up the JSNA and JHWS. To reinforce this duty NHS England has a duty to promote the use of these flexibilities by CCGs.

Section 75 Flexibilities

Pooled budgets

The pooling of budgets involves partner organisations contributing funds to a single pot, to be spent on agreed projects for designated services. They exist where a local authority and an NHS body combine resources and jointly commission or manage an integrated service. The idea is that, once a pooled budget is introduced the public will experience a seamless service with a single point of access for their health and social care needs. There are some areas that are particularly well suited to pooled budgets – for example, services for people with a learning disability.

Where a pooled budget exists, regulations for England and Wales require that the partners have written agreements setting out:

- the functions covered
- the aims agreed
- the funds that each partner will contribute
- which partner will act as the 'host' (i.e. which organisation will manage the budget and take responsibility for the accounts and auditing).

Aligned budgets

Aligned budgets can be either an informal or formal (using section 75 flexibilities) arrangement whereby partners align resources to meet agreed aims but have separate accountability for the respective funding streams. The management arrangements can be separate, joint or led by one partner but with joint performance monitoring arrangements against the objectives. An aligned budget can also be used as an interim stage to operating a pooled budget.

Lead commissioning

Under a lead commissioning arrangement, partners agree to delegate commissioning of a service to one lead organisation. As with pooled budgets, lead commissioning was made possible by section 31 of the *1999 Act* (now section 75 of the *NHS Act 2006*).

Integrated provision

Integrated provision involves partners joining together their staff, resources, and management structures so that the service is fully combined (or integrated) from managerial level to the front line. One partner acts as the host for the service to be provided. Again this way of working was made possible by section 31 of the *1999 Act* (now section 75 of the *NHS Act 2006*).

Government Grants

Government grants are available to the NHS for community-based projects run in conjunction with local authorities. Typically these grants are linked to regeneration and renewal programmes in deprived communities where a partnership board with representation from many elements of the local community (including NHS bodies) has successfully bid for and then managed the distribution of the grant. In terms of the financial framework for these projects, the structure is fairly straightforward – the grant is paid directly to the participating NHS body to cover the costs incurred.

Grants from the NHS to Local Authorities

NHS bodies have for many years been able to make grants to local authorities for the provision of health services (under sections 256/257 of the *NHS Act 2006* as amended*)*. This is broadly permissive and allows the transfer of capital or revenue resources for most health related functions (but not emergency ambulance services, surgery and other similar invasive treatments) and for most social services and housing functions. For example, a local authority operating a unit for people with learning difficulties may receive a grant from the NHS body to cover the provision of healthcare to the clients in the unit. Such grants must pay only for medical care and must not contribute towards the provision of social care. They must not involve the transfer of health functions to a local authority.

This power is still in place with CCGs or NHS England able to make payments to local authorities (or other bodies) towards expenditure on community services.

Grants from Local Authorities to the NHS

Section 76 of the *NHS Act 2006* (as amended) is a parallel provision to section 256 and allows the local authority to make payments to NHS bodies for the performance of prescribed functions. Again, this includes most hospital and community health services but not surgery, emergency ambulance services, etc. This power is still in place with local authorities able to make payments to NHS England or CCGs.

How Local Authorities are Financed

Local authority finance is entirely separate from the NHS and so is not discussed here. However, some NHS money does go to local authorities for two key purposes:

- health improvement – a ring fenced grant for local public health services is allocated to local authorities from 2013/14. Initially this is based on the amount that was spent in this area by primary care trusts in 2011/12. For 2013/14 the total budget is just under £2.7billon. For 2014/15 it will be just under £2.8 billion. In spending this money, local authorities must have regard to the *Public Health Outcomes Framework* and publish a Director of Public Health's annual report on the health of the local population
- social care priorities and to support collaboration/integration – in total £3billion is being transferred to local authorities over the current spending review period (2011/12 to 2014/15). In 2013/14 the allocation is £859m.

References and Further Reading

General information about local authorities – the Local Government Association:
www.local.gov.uk/

The Role of Local Authorities in Health Issues, Communities and Local Government Committee Report, March 2013:
www.publications.parliament.uk/pa/cm201213/cmselect/cmcomloc/694/69402.htm

The New Public Health Role of Local Authorities, Department of Health, 2012:
https://www.gov.uk/government/uploads/system/uploads/attachment_data/file/127045/Public-health-role-of-local-authorities-factsheet.pdf.pdf

Statutory guidance on JSNAs and JHWSs, Department of Health, 2013:
http://healthandcare.dh.gov.uk/jsnas-jhwss-guidance-published/

Operating principles for Health and Wellbeing Boards, NHS Confederation:
www.nhsconfed.org/Publications/Documents/Operating_principles_101011.pdf

For more on local HealthWatch: http://healthandcare.dh.gov.uk/what-is-healthwatch/

Public Health England: www.gov.uk/government/organisations/public-health-england

Public Health Outcomes Framework, Department of Health, 2012:
www.gov.uk/government/publications/public-health-outcomes-framework-update

NHS Act 2006: www.legislation.gov.uk/ukpga/2006/41/contents

The Community Care (Delayed Discharges etc) Act 2003:
www.legislation.gov.uk/ukpga/2003/5/contents

Public Health allocations to local authorities: https://www.gov.uk/government/publications/ring-fenced-public-health-grants-to-local-authorities-2013–14-and-2014–15

Chapter 9: NHS Finance – Who Does What?

The Role of the Regulators

> **Overview**
>
> This chapter looks at how the key sector wide regulators (Monitor, the Care Quality Commission and the National Institute for Health and Care Excellence) fit into the NHS, how they are structured, what they do and how they are financed. Please note that the focus is on the place of the regulators in the system, not on their approach to regulation – that is covered in chapter 12.
>
> To see where Monitor and the CQC fit into the NHS structure, look back at the diagram on page 16. NICE is not shown explicitly as it does not have a direct regulatory or funding relationship with healthcare providers – instead it falls within the Department of Health as one of its arm's length bodies (ALBs).

Monitor

What it is – constitution, structure and accountabilities

Monitor came into existence in 2004 as an executive non-departmental public body with a remit to authorise and regulate NHS foundation trusts (FTs). Although it is formally one of the Department of Health's 'arms' length bodies' (ALBs), it is independent of central government and directly accountable to Parliament rather than the Secretary of State for Health.

Monitor has a Board that consists of a Chairperson, non-executive directors (all appointed by the Secretary of State for Health) and executive directors. It also has an executive team and a number of other teams devoted to particular aspects of its role including a Medical Advisory Group that advises the Board on its strategy for improving the quality of care provided by FTs.

Like other ALBs, Monitor has a 'framework agreement' with the Department of Health which sets out its relationship and lines of accountability. It also submits a business plan to the Department for approval each year indicating how its objectives will be achieved and forecasting its financial performance. See chapter 3 for more about ALBs.

What Monitor does – roles and responsibilities

Pre 2012 Act

Monitor was established to authorise FTs and then regulate and monitor their performance against their terms of authorisation. Although Monitor's role has changed significantly as a result of the 2012 Act, it continues to play a role in assessing NHS trusts for FT status, and ensuring that FTs are 'financially viable and well-led, in terms of both quality and finances'.[1]

---

[1] Monitor website.

To qualify as an FT, applicant NHS trusts must meet stringent criteria set by the NHS Trust Development Authority (NHS TDA)[2] and pass Monitor's rigorous assessment process.

The FT assessment process

Before an NHS trust can apply to Monitor to be assessed, it must work with the NHS TDA to prepare a robust and credible application. It is the NHS TDA's responsibility (on behalf of the Secretary of State) to make sure that the trust is ready and able to apply to become an FT and it has developed a three stage approach that trusts must undergo.

Working with the NHS TDA – the Three Phases

- Diagnosis and due diligence – this involves establishing a baseline against which the FT application is built and includes a series of external reviews and self-assessments
- Development and application – this involves the trust submitting key documents to the NHS TDA and 'the testing and scrutiny of trust plans and personnel'[3]
- Assurance and approval – this is when the trust submits its final documents to the NHS TDA Board which decides whether or not the trust is ready to undergo a detailed assessment by Monitor

---

When the NHS TDA is satisfied that the trust is ready, its application is submitted to Monitor for its assessment.

Monitor's assessment process takes approximately three months and is described on Monitor's website as 'a robust and challenging process' that examines 'governance arrangements, financial viability, local accountability and performance against national standards and targets'. In essence there are three assessment criteria:

- **is the trust well governed?**
- **is the trust financially viable?**
- **is the trust legally constituted?**

The process involves due diligence, a 'board-to-board meeting' which is held midway through the assessment period and is designed to allow the applicant Board to 'demonstrate that it is aware of the risks facing the trust and provide details on how these risks can or have been managed and mitigated. This meeting also provides Monitor's Board with the opportunity to question the trust's non-executive directors to determine whether they have the skills required to effectively challenge the executive team.'[4]

---

[2] The NHS TDA was established under the 2012 Act to oversee all remaining NHS trusts and support them as they move towards foundation status.

[3] *Delivering High Quality Care for Patients: the Accountability Framework for NHS Trust Boards*, NHS TDA, April 2013.

[4] *Becoming an NHS Foundation Trust*, Monitor.

Applicants meeting the required standards are granted a licence that establishes them as an FT in the legal form of a public benefit entity. The licence also sets out the conditions under which the FT (and other licenced healthcare providers) must operate.

More information about the application process is available on the 'becoming a foundation trust' pages of Monitor's website.

Monitor's approach to regulation is looked at in chapter 12.

Post 2012 Act role

As mentioned above, Monitor's responsibilities have expanded as a result of the 2012 Act so that it is now the 'sector regulator for health'. Its overarching duty is to 'protect and promote the interests of people who use health care services … by promoting the provision of services which is economic, efficient and effective, and maintains or improves the quality of the services'.[5]

In practice, this means that Monitor is responsible for licensing all providers of NHS-funded care in England, including existing FTs (from April 2013), private and voluntary sector providers (from April 2014). If licence conditions are breached, Monitor can order the situation to be rectified and fine the provider if necessary. In extreme circumstances, Monitor has the power to remove directors and governors as well as revoke a provider's licence to operate.

In carrying out its licensing role, Monitor co-operates with the Care Quality Commission (CQC) which continues to be responsible for registering providers against 'essential levels of safety and quality'. The intention is that Monitor and the CQC will establish a single integrated process of licensing and registration.

In its new role as sector regulator, Monitor's core functions are:

- setting prices for NHS-funded care
- enabling integrated care
- safeguarding choice and preventing anti-competitive behaviour
- ensuring the continuity of services.

Monitor's Core Functions

Setting prices for NHS-funded services

The 2012 Act requires Monitor and NHS England to assume joint responsibility for setting prices. Monitor's focus is on designing the pricing methodology (based on information it collects from providers as required within the licence conditions) and using it to set prices whereas NHS England specifies the services to be priced (i.e. developing the pricing

---

[5] Monitor's new role: www.monitor-nhsft.gov.uk/monitors-new-role.

structure) and agreeing these with Monitor. Once agreed by Monitor and NHS England, prices are published in a document called the National Tariff. It is expected that this approach will start for the 2014/15 tariff.

Clinical commissioning groups (CCGs) are consulted on the underlying methodology used to set the tariff and can raise objections. Monitor can alter tariffs but only in relation to a new category of service – namely those services that are 'designated as subject to additional regulation' which will be identified in providers' licences as 'commissioner requested services'. These are services which, if lost, would result in 'material damage to patients' – essential services for which there is no immediate alternative or re-provision if they cease. However, if the tariff is altered, the regulator must pay heed to a number of duties – to protect patients and the public through competition where appropriate and regulation where necessary; to promote efficiency and to adhere to European Union rules (ensuring providers do not gain an unfair competitive advantage or the tariff change does not constitute unlawful state aid).

Enabling integrated care

Monitor has a general duty to consider how it can enable or facilitate integrated care to help improve the quality of services or provide better access for patients. This will include working with others (and in particular, commissioners) to remove any barriers.

Safeguarding choice and preventing anti-competitive behaviour

Although CCGs and NHS England will decide where competition is used, Monitor makes sure that it is fair and operates in the interests of patients. To do this, Monitor has powers such as those exercised by OFCOM and OFGEM to apply competition law to prevent anti-competitive behaviour, initially only for healthcare providers (public and private) but eventually to include providers of adult social care. To enable it to carry out this role, Monitor has 'concurrent powers' with the Office of Fair Trading (OFT) to apply the Competition Act 1998 – this allows either Monitor or the OFT to investigate provider practices that might restrict competition. Monitor can also set specific licence conditions if it can demonstrate that this will protect competition; conduct market reviews where competition is not functioning properly and refer markets to the Competition Commission for investigation.

Monitor also protects patients' ability to choose by tackling specific abuses and restrictions that act against patients' interests and ensuring that (amongst other things) there is a fair playing field for all providers. Monitor can also issue regulations to govern commissioners' procurement activities and 'parties with a legitimate interest' can complain to Monitor if they believe commissioners have broken these rules. Commissioners and providers can seek judicial review if they are dissatisfied with Monitor's decisions.

Supporting the continuity of services

Monitor is required under the 2012 Act to ensure that if a healthcare provider fails, patients will still be able to access the care they need. This is the so-called 'continuity of service regime' – although the primary responsibility for ensuring that services are available lies with commissioners (supported by NHS England), Monitor has a duty to 'prevent providers from taking actions that could undermine their continued ability to deliver services'. Monitor can also help providers who are having problems (for example, by requiring them to appoint turnaround experts to help avoid failure). In exceptional circumstances, Monitor can appoint a 'trust special administrator' to take control of the provider's business and work with commissioners to make sure that patients can still access services. Where a provider is in financial difficulty, Monitor has a duty to make available a source of finance to cover the costs of administration, via a risk pool arrangement – a fund that is built up via levies on providers and commissioners. However, there is an overarching principle in the 2012 Act that additional regulation will not apply unless 'commissioners can demonstrate that the loss of a particular service... would result in material damage to patients.'

Monitor will retain its regulator role in relation to the financial and governance performance of FTs until 2016. After that, the intention is that governing bodies 'self-regulate' their organisations.

How Monitor is Financed

Monitor is funded through government grant-in-aid from the Department of Health.

Care Quality Commission (CQC)

What it is – constitution, structure and accountabilities

The Care Quality Commission began operating on 1 April 2009 as the independent regulator of health and adult social care in England. It is an executive non-departmental public body and was established to regulate the essential standards of quality and safety, which are set out in the *Health and Social Care Act 2008*.

Although (like Monitor) it is formally an ALB of the Department of Health, the CQC is independent of central government and directly accountable to Parliament. However (as with Monitor and all ALBs), the CQC does have a 'framework agreement' with the Department of Health which sets out its relationship and lines of accountability. It also submits a business plan to the Department for approval each year indicating how its objectives will be achieved and forecasting its financial performance. See chapter 3 for more about ALBs.

The CQC has a Board and an executive team – see the website for details.

What it does – roles and responsibilities

The CQC was given a range of legal powers and duties as part of the 2008 Act, these include:

CQC Powers and Duties (2008 Act)

- Registering providers of healthcare and social care to ensure they are meeting the essential standards of quality and safety
- Monitoring how providers comply with the standards by gathering information and inspecting them when the CQC think it is needed
- Using enforcement powers, such as fines and public warnings and closing down services, if services drop below the essential standards and particularly if the CQC think that people's rights or safety are at risk
- Acting to protect patients whose rights are restricted under the Mental Health Act
- Promoting improvement in services by conducting regular reviews of how well those who arrange and provide services locally are performing
- Carrying out special reviews of particular types of services and pathways of care, or investigations on areas where the CQC has concerns about quality and safety
- Seeking the views of people who use services and involving them in the CQC's work
- Telling people about the quality of their local care services to help providers and commissioners of services to learn from each other about what works best and where improvement is needed, and help to shape national policy

As a result of the 2012 Act, the CQC now has additional responsibilities – these include:

CQC Responsibilities (2012 Act)

- HealthWatch England – this is a new national body that has been established to enable the views of people who use NHS and social care services to influence national policy, advice and guidance. It is constituted as a statutory committee of the CQC and its Chairperson is a CQC non-executive director. Its role is to provide leadership, guidance and support to local HealthWatch organisations (see chapter 8) and advise the Secretary of State, NHS England, Monitor and local authorities. HealthWatch England is funded as part of the Department of Health's grant in aid to the CQC and must make an annual report to Parliament
- The integration of the National Information Governance Board for Health and Social Care into the CQC
- In the longer term the integration of certain functions of the Human Fertilisation and Embryology Authority and the Human Tissue Authority into the CQC

How the CQC is financed

The CQC is funded through a combination of registration fee income and government grant-in-aid from the Department of Health.

The National Institute for Health and Care Excellence (NICE)

What it is – constitution, structure and accountabilities

NICE was set up in 1999 as the National Institute for Clinical Excellence with the aim of reducing variation in the availability and quality of NHS treatments and care. In 2005, NICE merged with the Health Development Agency and began developing public health guidance – its full name changed to the National Institute for Health and Clinical Excellence. In April 2013, NICE took on responsibility for developing guidance and quality standards in social care resulting in a further name change.

In constitutional terms NICE is an executive non-departmental public body (prior to the 2012 Act it was a special health authority). This means that it is an ALB of the Department of Health with a framework agreement that sets out its relationship and lines of accountability. It also submits a business plan to the Department for approval each year indicating how its objectives will be achieved and forecasting its financial performance. See chapter 3 for more about ALBs.

NICE has a Board comprising non-executive and executive directors and a senior management team.

What NICE does – roles and responsibilities

NICE's key role is 'to improve outcomes for people using the NHS and other public health and social care services'.[6] This includes producing:

- evidence-based guidance and other products to help 'resolve uncertainty about which medicines, treatments, procedures and devices represent the best quality care and which offer the best value for money for the NHS'
- 'public health guidance recommending best ways to encourage healthy living, promote wellbeing and prevent disease'.

NICE also has a library of quality standards and metrics that are used in the *NHS Outcomes Framework*, the *Clinical Commissioning Group Outcomes Indicator Set* and to inform payment mechanisms and incentive schemes such as the Quality and Outcomes Framework (QOF) and Commissioning for Quality and Innovation (CQUIN) payment framework.

These quality standards are 'a set of specific, concise statements and associated measures. They set out aspirational, but achievable, markers of high-quality, cost-effective patient care, covering the treatment and prevention of different diseases and conditions'. Standards already exist for a wide range of conditions and interventions including mental health and respiratory medicine.

The *Health and Social Care Act 2012* sets out a new responsibility for NICE to develop quality standards and other guidance for social care in England.

How NICE is financed

NICE is funded primarily by grant-in-aid from the Department of Health with small amounts of income from other government departments and NHS bodies.

---

[6] NICE website.

References and Further Reading

General information about Monitor (including membership details of its Board, executive team and Medical Advisory Group): www.monitor-nhsft.gov.uk/about-monitor/who-we-are

Delivering High Quality Care for Patients: the Accountability Framework for NHS Trust Boards, NHS TDA, April 2013:
www.ntda.nhs.uk/wp-content/uploads/2012/04/framework_050413_web.pdf

Becoming a Foundation Trust, Monitor:
www.monitor-nhsft.gov.uk/becoming-nhs-foundation-trust

Monitor's new role as sector regulator of NHS-funded healthcare services:
www.monitor-nhsft.gov.uk/monitors-new-role

Regulations on procurement, patient choice and competition, Department of Health, 2013:
https://www.gov.uk/government/publications/regulations-on-procurement-patient-choice-and-competition

Information about Monitor's failure regime and trust special administrators:
www.monitor-nhsft.gov.uk/home/news-events-and-publications/latest-press-releases/monitor-takes-new-powers-protect-patient-ser

Care Quality Commission: www.cqc.org.uk/

HealthWatch England: http://healthandcare.dh.gov.uk/what-is-healthwatch/

NICE: www.nice.org.uk/

Details of NICE's work and links to key documents:
www.nice.org.uk/aboutnice/whatwedo/what_we_do.jsp

NHS Outcomes Framework, Department of Health, 2013:
www.gov.uk/government/publications/nhs-outcomes-framework-2013-to-2014

Information about the Quality and Outcomes Framework (QOF): www.nhsemployers.org/
PayAndContracts/GeneralMedicalServicesContract/QOF/Pages/QualityOutcomesFramework.aspx

Information about the Commissioning for Quality and Innovation (CQUIN) Payment Framework:
www.gov.uk/government/publications/using-the-commissioning-for-quality-and-innovation-cquin-payment-framework-guidance-on-new-national-goals-for-2012–13

Chapter 10: How the NHS is Financed

Overview

Health spending has always been a topic of political and public interest and in the last decade spending on health increased at a significantly higher rate than many other government programmes. Even now, in a time of austerity, health funding has been protected.

This chapter focuses on how resources are allocated nationally for the NHS and how they are divided up amongst the different areas of health spending. It also gives an idea of the scale of UK spending on health compared with other countries.

UK Spending Levels

The Organisation for Economic Cooperation and Development (OECD) health data for 2012 shows that during 2010, the United Kingdom spent 9.6% of gross domestic product (GDP)[1] on health. This compared with an average across the 30 OECD countries of 9.5% although this figure is made up of national spending in excess of the average – for example, 11.6% in France and 17.6% in the USA. The data also indicated that in 2010, 83.2% of total spending on health in the UK came from general government expenditure – well above the average for OECD countries of 72.2%. Although the percentage of GDP spent on health in the UK has been rising steadily since 2002/03 when it was 7.7%, constraints on public spending following the economic downturn in 2008/09 mean that spending is now expected to plateau.

The Role of the Treasury

The responsibility for allocating and managing the finances of national government lies with the Chancellor of the Exchequer, who leads the Treasury. To promote better planning of public spending the Treasury undertakes periodic spending reviews to set 'departmental expenditure limits' (DELs) for each government department. DELs usually cover a period of three years.

There have been six spending reviews since they were first introduced in 1998. These spending reviews are themselves reviewed twice a year – in the budget and the pre-budget report, where the Government sets out how it will finance its spending commitments and makes any necessary or technical adjustments to its spending plans. The spending review in October 2010 set out the Coalition Government's departmental spending plans for the next four years – up until 2014/15. The next spending review takes place in June 2013.

Public expenditure falls into one of two categories:

- DEL spending, which is planned and controlled on a three year basis in spending reviews

---

[1] GDP is the total money value of all final goods and services produced in an economy during a year.

- annually managed expenditure (AME), which is expenditure that cannot reasonably be subject to firm, multi-year limits in the same way as DEL. Examples of such spending are social security benefits which are subject to fluctuation depending on the level of unemployment.

Together, DEL plus AME sum to 'total managed expenditure' (TME).

A key issue for any government is the relative level of public spending compared to national wealth. Relative to GDP (which itself fluctuates from year to year), UK public spending since 1970 has varied from 49.7% in 1975/76 to 36.3% in 1999/00. The predicted position for 2012/13 is 39%.

The Treasury allocates DELs for revenue and capital spending. Revenue spending is for day-to-day items such as salaries and running costs; capital spending is for buying larger items such as buildings and equipment, which have a usable life of over one year.

The Treasury's 2010 spending review resulted in the following pattern of allocations of revenue and capital DELs to government departments:

Total Department Programme and Administration Budgets – revenue (or 'resource') DEL excluding depreciation and capital				
	2011/12 £bn	2012/13 £bn	2013/14 £bn	2014/15 £bn
NHS (Health)	101.5	104.0	106.9	109.8
Education	51.2	52.1	52.9	53.9
Energy and Climate Change	1.5	1.4	1.3	1.0
Communities and Local Government	28.1	26.1	25.8	24.1
Defence	24.9	25.2	24.9	24.7
Home Office	8.9	8.5	8.1	7.8
Foreign and Commonwealth Office	1.5	1.5	1.4	1.2
Justice	8.1	7.7	7.4	7.0
Business, Innovation and Skills	16.5	15.6	14.7	13.7
Transport	5.3	5.0	5.0	4.4
International Development	6.7	7.2	9.4	9.4
Work and Pensions	7.6	7.4	7.4	7.6
Scotland	24.8	25.1	25.3	25.4
Wales	13.3	13.3	13.5	13.5
Northern Ireland	9.4	9.4	9.5	9.5
Other Departments and Reserve	17.4	17.4	17.4	15.9
TOTAL DEL	**326.7**	**326.9**	**330.9**	**328.9**

Source: Spending Review 2010, HM Treasury.

Total Department Capital DEL

	2011/12 £bn	2012/13 £bn	2013/14 £bn	2014/15 £bn
NHS (Health)	4.4	4.4	4.4	4.6
Education	4.9	4.2	3.3	3.4
Energy and Climate Change	1.5	2.0	2.2	2.7
Communities and Local Government	3.3	2.3	1.8	2.0
Defence	8.9	9.1	9.2	8.7
Home Office	0.5	0.5	0.4	0.5
Foreign and Commonwealth Office	0.1	0.1	0.1	0.1
Justice	0.4	0.3	0.3	0.3
Business, Innovation and Skills	1.2	1.1	0.8	1.0
Transport	7.7	8.1	7.5	7.5
International Development	1.4	1.6	1.9	2.0
Work and Pensions	0.2	0.3	0.4	0.2
Scotland	2.5	2.5	2.2	2.3
Wales	1.3	1.2	1.1	1.1
Northern Ireland	0.9	0.9	0.8	0.8
Other Departments and Reserves	4.3	3.2	2.8	3.0
TOTAL Capital DEL	**43.5**	**41.8**	**39.2**	**40.2**

Source: Spending Review 2010, HM Treasury.

For the NHS in England the position over the spending review period (including percentage growth rates) is summarised in the table that follows:

The NHS in England

	2011/12 £bn	2012/13 £bn	2013/14 £bn	2014/15 £bn
DEL Settlement i.e. the sum of resource DEL (excluding depreciation) and capital DEL				
NHS (Health) REVENUE	101.50	104.00	106.90	109.80
annual growth	2.8%	2.5%	2.8%	2.7%
NHS (Health) CAPITAL	4.40	4.40	4.40	4.60
annual growth	−13.7%	0.0%	0.0%	4.5%
NHS (Health) TOTAL	**105.90**	**108.40**	**111.30**	**114.40**
annual growth	**2.0%**	**2.4%**	**2.7%**	**2.8%**
GDP deflator to take account of inflation	1.9%	2.3%	2.6%	2.7%
Real growth	0.1%	0.1%	0.1%	0.1%

Source: Spending Review 2010, HM Treasury

Each year when the Chancellor announces the budget these figures are reviewed and (where necessary) adjusted. In the 2013 budget the impact on health spending is shown below – as you can see, the estimate for 2012/13 indicates an underspend on both revenue and capital.

Revenue and Capital DEL for the NHS			
	2012/13 (estimate) £bn	2013/14 (plan) £bn	2014/15 (plan) £bn
NHS (Health) – revenue	102.9	106.9	109.8
NHS (Health) – capital	3.7	4.4	4.6
NHS total	106.6	111.3	114.4

Source: Budget 2013, HM Treasury.

Funding for health services in other UK nations is included in the separate Northern Ireland, Scottish and Welsh block grants. Any changes in planned spending in the NHS in England are matched by relative increases within these block grants. However, the individual administrations may spend less or more than these amounts on health services depending on their own priorities.

The Role of the Department of Health

The Department of Health decides how the funding it receives from the Treasury is allocated in England. Health and social services in Northern Ireland, Scotland and Wales are the responsibility of devolved administrations (see chapters 20 to 22).

Most of the total NHS settlement (over 80%) is allocated to NHS England which keeps around 20% for its own commissioning responsibilities and running costs and allocates the rest to clinical commissioning groups (CCGs).

However, the Department retains part of the allocation to meet:

- its own running costs
- the costs of various central health and miscellaneous services (CHMS) – for example, some centrally administered services and projects managed centrally for the benefit of the NHS (such as clinical negligence); a range of statutory and other arm's length bodies funded centrally (for example, the NHS Business Services Authority, Health Education England and the NHS Trust Development Authority – see chapter 3 for details)
- the costs of public health spending – this is covered by a separate ring fenced budget (from the Department of Health's allocation) that is passed to and managed by local authorities and Public Health England (an executive agency within the Department – see chapter 3).

The Role of NHS England

From 2013/14 NHS England is responsible for using the funding it receives from the Department to deliver the mandate that it agrees annually. In practice this means NHS England's allocation has to fund the costs of:

- running NHS England, its area teams, local professional networks, clinical senates and networks
- its direct commissioning activities – including the primary medical services provided by GPs, dentists, community pharmacists and opticians; specialised services; offender and military healthcare
- CCG commissioning
- running CCGs (known as the 'running cost allowance')
- some services that are commissioned by local authorities.

For 2013/14 the total revenue budget allocated to NHS England to deliver the Mandate is £95.6 billion[2] with £63.4 billion (just over 66% of the total) allocated to CCGs and £0.9bn to local authorities. The way in which the total budget is split is shown below:

Recipient	Area of Spend	How Much? (£billion)
NHS England	See table that follows	30.0
CCGs	Local services commissioned for their populations	63.4
CCGs	Running costs	1.3
Local authorities	Services that benefit health and social care	0.9
Total		**95.6**

NHS England's own allocation for 2013/14 of £30 billion is split as follows:

Area of Spend	How Much? (£ billion)
Commissioning of specialised healthcare, primary care, military and offender services	25.4
Public health on behalf of Public Health England (immunisation, screening and health visiting)	1.8
Surplus carry forward from primary care trusts (PCTs) and strategic health authorities (SHAs) to be allocated to CCGs and NHS England for future investment	1.2
Central health programmes (for example, clinical excellence awards and support for PFI schemes)	1.0
Technical accounting adjustments	0.7
Total (N.B. does not total to 30 due to roundings)	**30.1**

---

[2] NHS England also has a capital budget for 2013/14 of £200m.

The allocations made to NHS England and by it to CCGs are resource and cash-limited and they have a statutory duty not to exceed these limits (see chapter 11 for more on financial duties).

The allocations to CCGs are then used by them to commission the majority of NHS services for their patients including:

- planned hospital care
- rehabilitative care
- urgent and emergency services including out-of-hours services
- community health services
- maternity services
- mental health services
- learning disabilities services.

In practice, this means that CCGs agree contracts with 'any qualified providers' of acute, specialist and mental health care – see chapter 5 for more about CCGs.

CCG Allocations

For the first year of the new funding system (2013/14), resources have been allocated to each individual CCG based on PCT expenditure plans for 2012/13 with the result that all CCGs have received 'an above real terms uniform increase in funding'.[3]

This means that the 2013/14 allocations are effectively based on the approach that was in use for many years to make allocations to PCTs. It is expected that a similar approach will be used in future although the formula initially proposed by the Advisory Committee on Resource Allocation (ACRA) has not been accepted by NHS England as 'it is concerned that use of the formula on its own to redistribute funding would predominantly have resulted in higher growth for areas that already have the best health outcomes compared to those with the worst. On the face of it, this appears inconsistent with NHS England's public purpose to improve health outcomes for all patients and citizens and reduce health inequalities. It will therefore conduct an urgent, fundamental review of the approach to allocations, drawing on the expert advice of ACRA and involving all partners whose functions impact on outcomes and inequalities. It will be completed in time for initial conclusions to inform 2014/15 allocations.'[4]

If you would like to know more about how the 'old' PCT allocation process (including the 'weighted capitation formula') worked, see Appendix 1.

Once a CCG has been notified of its allocation for the forthcoming year, it plans how to use the funding across the full range of services that it commissions with the overall aim of improving the health and wellbeing of its population. A CCG commissions services from a range of providers including NHS trusts and foundation trusts, the private and voluntary sectors (see chapter 16 for more on commissioning).

---

[3] *Everyone Counts: Planning for Patients 2013/14*, NHS England, 2012.
[4] *Everyone Counts: Planning for Patients 2013/14*, NHS England, 2012.

NHS and Foundation Trusts

The majority of community, acute, specialist and mental healthcare in England is provided by NHS trusts or NHS foundation trusts. These trusts meet the costs of providing healthcare services (staff salaries are normally the largest element) and receive income from CCGs (and for some services, from NHS England) via standard contracts that specify the quantity, quality and price of services to be provided (for activity covered by payment by results (PbR), the unit price is dictated by a nationally set tariff). Each CCG (or NHS England) is responsible for meeting the cost of services provided to its population in line with the contract's terms. CCGs, NHS England and providers are responsible for ensuring that patient treatments are clinically appropriate and provided in a cost effective way.

Trusts also receive some income from other sources such as private patient income, research, hosting services, car park receipts and leasing of buildings. In addition, some trusts get substantial sums from the monies earmarked in the centrally held budgets referred to earlier in this chapter, in particular to cover the education and training of clinical staff. From April 2013, these funding flows are governed by Health Education England (HEE) and a new education tariff system is being put into place.

Many trusts also have access to funds donated on a charitable basis – for example, by members of the public. However these can be used only for the purpose for which they were given – for more about charitable funds see chapter 19.

Primary Care Services

The majority of primary care services are provided by independent contractors such as general medical practitioners (GPs), general dental practitioners (GDPs), pharmacists and ophthalmic practitioners. Whilst they are an integral part of the NHS, these contractors operate as small businesses that contract with the NHS to provide primary care services. Contracts are designed to reward the quality of treatment.

NHS England pays primary care service providers according to nationally negotiated contracts – although extensions to the basic contract are negotiated locally. For example, GP practices receive a global sum to cover the provision of core services to their registered practice list and additional 'quality' payments for achieving goals set out in the quality and outcomes framework (QOF).

The interface between primary and secondary care is not always clear and GPs with specialist interests are increasingly playing a significant part in delivering patient care outside of the traditional hospital routes.

See chapter 6 for more on primary care services.

What is the Money Spent on?

Since 2003/04, the Department of Health has collected information about how the billions invested in the NHS are spent and what is achieved for that investment. The idea is to collect information in a consistent manner about the clinical areas (or 'programme budgets') in which NHS resources are being spent.

The main aims of programme budgeting are to provide a:

- way of monitoring where NHS resources are invested
- way of assisting in evaluating the effectiveness of the pattern of resource deployment
- tool to support and improve the process for identifying the most effective way of commissioning NHS services for the future.

The latest figures (in £ billion) for 2011/12 across programme budget categories are shown below in diagrammatic form:

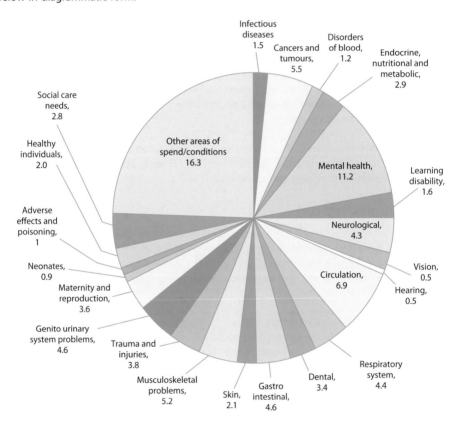

Of the programme areas identified (excluding 'other'), spending on mental health accounts for the largest single proportion of NHS spending at just under 12% of the total. Note that the 'other' category includes expenditure on primary medical services.

Programme budgeting now includes a breakdown of expenditure by care setting to help commissioners understand their expenditure in more detail. NHS England will continue work to develop the collection further to provide CCGs with more useful and meaningful information on spending patterns.

Key Learning Points

- The UK spends 9.6% of GDP on health – just above the OECD average
- The Treasury decides how much money each government department receives based on spending reviews
- Money is allocated for both day-to-day (revenue) and capital spending
- The Department of Health decides how the budget is used with over 80% going to NHS England; there is also a ring fenced budget for public health
- The Department keeps some money for central services and arms' length bodies such as Public Health England and Health Education England
- NHS England allocates the bulk of the money it receives to CCGs but keeps some to fund its own direct commissioning functions and running costs
- CCG allocations were based initially on PCT funding levels but a new formula will be used from 2014/15
- NHS and foundation trusts receive the bulk of their income via contracts with CCGs and NHS England; other sources include income from private patients
- Primary care services are provided predominantly by independent contractors who receive income via contracts agreed with NHS England
- Programme budgeting information is collected each year and shows how NHS money is spent.

References and Further Reading

Health Data 2012, Organisation for Economic Cooperation and Development (OECD): www.oecd.org/health/health-systems/oecdhealthdata2012.htm

Spending Review 2010, HM Treasury: www.hm-treasury.gov.uk/spend_index.htm

Budget 2013, HM Treasury: www.hm-treasury.gov.uk/budget2013_documents.htm

The NHS Mandate: www.gov.uk/government/publications/the-nhs-mandate

NHS England allocations announcement for 2013/14: www.england.nhs.uk/allocations-2013–14/

Everyone Counts: Planning for Patients 2013/14, NHS England, 2012: www.england.nhs.uk/everyonecounts/

Health Education England: http://hee.nhs.uk/

2011/12 programme budgeting information, NHS Networks: www.networks.nhs.uk/nhs-networks/health-investment-network/news/2011-12-programme-budgeting-data-now-available

Programme budgeting information: https://www.gov.uk/government/publications/overview-of-the-programme-budgeting-methodology

Chapter 11: How NHS Organisations Demonstrate Financial Accountability

> ## Overview
>
> This chapter looks at the key financial and performance reporting mechanisms that NHS organisations use to demonstrate accountability in financial terms. Its primary focus is on external reporting requirements but there is also a section on internal reporting to budget holders and governing bodies.

External Reporting

Statutory requirements

All NHS bodies have a statutory duty to produce an annual report and accounts[1] with the form and content directed by the Secretary of State for Health (for NHS England and NHS trusts); NHS England (for clinical commissioning groups) and the independent regulator, Monitor (for foundation trusts).

The production of the annual accounts is the principal means by which NHS bodies discharge their accountability to taxpayers and users of services for their stewardship of public money.

Accounting framework

NHS bodies must follow international financial reporting standards (IFRS) as issued or endorsed by the International Accounting Standards Board (IASB) for the preparation of accounts. These standards are intended to provide a framework for good practice, the common disclosure of information and a benchmark against which an organisation's audited accounts are judged.

Although NHS bodies must adhere to IFRSs, the Government has the final say on how these standards are applied to the public sector (including NHS bodies) with details set out in the Treasury's *Financial Reporting Manual*. This is because IFRSs are written with profit making organisations in mind and therefore some interpretation is required to allow them to be applied consistently to public sector bodies where profit making is not as relevant.

At present, the Department of Health also produces a *Manual for Accounts* that is consistent with the requirements of the *Financial Reporting Manual* and which non-foundation NHS bodies are required to follow. Monitor produces a similar manual for FTs, called the *NHS*

---

[1] For CCGs this duty is set out in *the Health and Social Care Act 2012*, part 1, section 26, sub section 14Z15 and schedule 2, paragraph 17 (2). For NHS trusts, the relevant legislation is section 232 and paragraph 3(1) of schedule 15 of the *NHS Act 2006* as amended by part 4, section 154 of the 2012 Act; for NHS foundation trusts (FTs) the relevant legislation is section 30 and paragraph 25(1) of schedule 7 of the *NHS Act 2006* as amended by part 4, section 154 of the 2012 Act.

Foundation Trust Annual Reporting Manual. NHS England is responsible for producing comparable guidance for clinical commissioning groups (CCGs) with the first such manual expected later in 2013 for CCGs to use when preparing their 2013/14 accounts. These manuals are updated each year and include a summary of the relevant accounting standards. However, if an organisation needs a more detailed understanding of a particular aspect it should refer to the relevant standard in full.

Annual accounts

The Department's *Manual for Accounts*, the *NHS Foundation Trust Annual Reporting Manual* and NHS England's guidance for CCGs specify the format of the annual accounts which differs slightly depending upon the type of NHS body concerned. However, the main elements are shown below:

What the Annual Accounts Contain

The **foreword** to the accounts

The **four primary statements**:

- statement of comprehensive income or statement of comprehensive net expenditure
- statement of financial position
- statement of changes in taxpayers' equity
- statement of cash flows.

Notes to the accounts

Statements and certificates: directors' statement of responsibilities; the accounting (or accountable) officer's statement of responsibilities; the annual governance statement (see below); and the auditors' report.

Annual governance statement

NHS organisations produce an annual governance statement that forms part of the annual accounts. This statement focuses on the stewardship of the organisation and draws together 'position statements and evidence on governance, risk management and control, to provide a more coherent and consistent reporting mechanism'.[2] Although there is no prescribed format the statement must cover a number of areas including:

- scope of the organisation's Accounting (or Accountable) Officer's responsibilities
- information about the organisation's governance framework
- a description of how risk is assessed and managed
- information about how the risk and control framework works

---

[2] 2012/13 governance statement guidance, Department of Health, 2013.

- a review of the effectiveness of risk management and internal control
- any significant control issues and how they are being addressed.

Each year, the Department of Health issues guidance for NHS organisations to use when preparing their governance statement. There is also a useful explanation of what governance statements are designed to achieve in Annex 3.1 of the Treasury's publication *Managing Public Money*.

Quality accounts

Since April 2010, all providers of acute care (including mental health, ambulance and disability learning trusts) are required to produce an annual quality account (also referred to as a quality report) in line with the statutory requirement set out in the *Health Act 2009*. The aim is to 'enhance accountability to the public and engage the leaders of an organisation in their quality improvement agenda' by reporting the continuous improvement in the quality of the services provided. From April 2013, a core set of quality indicators must be included in all NHS bodies' quality accounts to support the mandate agreed between the Government and NHS England. The prescribed indicators for 2012/13 are set out in statutory instruments supporting the 2009 Act[3] and guidance issued by the Department of Health.[4]

Quality accounts must be shared for comment with the relevant NHS England area team, 'dominant' CCG and local health and wellbeing board. The final agreed quality account must be sent to the Secretary of State and made available via the NHS Choices website.

Parts of the quality accounts are subject to review by auditors as set out in guidance issued by Monitor and the Audit Commission.

What Quality Accounts Include

- An overall statement of accountability from the Board
- Three to five priorities for improvement
- A review of quality performance (including at least three indicators from each of the three 'domains of quality' – safety, effectiveness and patient experience)
- Research and innovation
- What others say about the provider
- Data quality

Annual report

As mentioned above, all NHS bodies are required to produce an annual report which must be published with the full set of audited accounts. The annual report is primarily a narrative

---

[3] *National Health Service (Quality Accounts) Regulations 2010, National Health Service (Quality Accounts) Amendment Regulations 2011.*
[4] *Changes to Quality Accounts reporting arrangements*, Department of Health, 2013.

document similar to the directors' report and the remuneration report described in the *Companies Act*, but with additional information reflecting the NHS body's position in the community. The report gives an account of the body's activities and performance over the last financial year.

Although the overall layout of the annual report is at each NHS body's discretion, there are mandatory items that must be included – these are Companies Act and HM Treasury requirements which apply to NHS bodies. These are set out in the *Manual for Accounts/NHS Foundation Trust Annual Reporting Manual*/NHS England guidance for CCGs. Organisations also use the annual report as an opportunity to set out their achievements in the year and highlight the challenges ahead.

The annual report must be published along with the audited accounts (see below) as one document and approved by the governing body prior to being presented at a public meeting. For non-foundation organisations, this meeting must be held before 30 September following the end of the relevant financial year.

NHS bodies can also prepare and make available an annual report and summary financial statements – however, this is additional to the full annual report and accounts.

For FTs, the annual report and accounts must be approved by the Board of Directors prior to submission to Monitor. FTs must lay their report and accounts (the full accounts – not summary financial statements) before Parliament themselves prior to the summer recess. The annual report and accounts must also be presented to a meeting of the FT's Council of Governors. This meeting should be convened within a reasonable timescale after the end of the financial year, but must not be before the FT has laid the annual report and accounts before Parliament.

CCGs must produce an annual report following the format required by NHS England,[5] which must be both published and presented to the public. The annual report must show how the CCG has contributed to the relevant health and wellbeing strategy, and how it has:

* improved the quality of services
* reduced health inequalities
* involved and consulted with the public.

Audit

As mentioned above, the NHS organisation's annual accounts must be audited prior to their adoption by the governing body and publication. To be able to carry out their audit, auditors must be given a copy of the annual report along with the accounts and working papers at the start of the audit so that they have sufficient time to carry out the required work before the completion of the auditor's opinion. The annual report is read by auditors to ensure consistency with the annual accounts and their knowledge of the NHS body. Some parts of the

---

[5] Section 14Z15 of the *NHS Act 2006* as inserted by s26 of the *Health and Social Care Act 2012.*

annual report are subject to audit in the same way as the accounts – for example, elements of the remuneration report. After the accounts have been audited and any necessary amendments made, the governing body is required to formally adopt the accounts. The certificates are signed at the same time. The auditor then signs the audit report.

Timetable

The *Manual for Accounts/FT Annual Reporting Manual*/NHS England guidance for CCGs also set out the timetable for completion of the accounts and audit. This timetable has been brought forward over recent years and for 2013/14, draft accounts had to be submitted for audit by 22 April 2013 with an audit deadline of 10 June 2013. FTs currently work to a slightly shorter timescale – although their draft accounts had to be completed to the same deadline (22 April 2013), they had to submit audited accounts by 30 May 2013.

Operating and financial review

It is considered best practice for public sector organisations to produce an operating and financial review (OFR) but it is not mandatory. If an OFR is produced, its content is decided by the organisation and should include details of performance that are not reported in the annual accounts including useful non-financial and financial information.

Commissioning plans

Each CCG must prepare an annual commissioning plan[6] that sets out how it proposes to 'exercise its functions' – this includes how it plans to spend the funding received on buying healthcare for its constituent practices' patients. These plans must be published and submitted to NHS England and all relevant health and wellbeing boards before the start of the financial year to which they relate. A CCG must also have detailed financial plans that are consistent with its commissioning plan.

Monitoring reports

As well as preparing the statutory annual accounts, NHS trusts are required to submit financial monitoring and accounts (FMA) forms to the Department of Health throughout the year. FMA forms are consistent with the annual accounts, but contain slightly different information and are used by the Department to monitor financial performance throughout the year and, at the year end, prepare the summarised accounts for each type of NHS body and the Department's own resource account.[7]

FTs have to complete similar monitoring reports for Monitor throughout the year. At the year end, FTs are required to complete consolidation schedules which are consistent with their annual accounts and provide additional information which is used by Monitor to produce a summary of FT accounts which are then included in the Department of Health's consolidated accounts.

---

[6] Section 14Z11 of the *NHS Act 2006* as inserted by s26 of the *Health and Social Care Act 2012*.
[7] The resource account shows how the money allocated to the Department has been spent.

In the case of CCGs, the 2012 Act (schedule 1A paragraph 18) requires them to provide financial information to NHS England throughout the financial year which is used to monitor their financial performance.

The use of these FMA forms, consolidation schedules and regular financial information also facilitates the preparation of whole of government accounts (WGA) – the consolidated set of financial statements for the UK public sector.

Trusts are also subject to monthly workforce monitoring which includes an analysis of pay expenditure.

Financial Performance Targets

As well as the statutory requirement to produce annual accounts and reports, NHS bodies are subject to a range of statutory and departmental financial targets. The targets and their nature vary according to the type of NHS body – those that apply in 2013/14 are set out below.

NHS England

NHS England's key statutory financial duty is to ensure that in each financial year total spending on health does not exceed the income received. NHS England must ensure that:

- total capital resource used in a financial year does not exceed the amount specified by the Secretary of State (known as the capital resource limit or CRL)
- total revenue resource used in a financial year does not exceed the amount specified by the Secretary of State (known as the revenue resource limit or RRL).

NHS England is also enabled by the 2012 Act to use some of the funding it receives to establish a contingency fund which can be used to help discharge its functions or to help CCGs discharge their functions.

In relation to revenue and capital resource limits, NHS England's Chief Executive (the Accounting Officer) is held to account by the Department of Health. NHS England is also required to prepare a consolidated annual account for all CCGs which is a key element in the Department of Health's overall resource account.

Clinical commissioning groups

To be able to fulfil its statutory requirements, NHS England holds CCGs to account for their stewardship of resources and outcomes achieved.

The key financial duty as set out in section 27 of the 2012 Act is that each CCG must not spend more in a year than it receives. In addition, in relation to both revenue and capital resources, each CCG must not spend more than an amount specified by direction of NHS England. In other words each CCG must not exceed its revenue and capital resource limits.

As mentioned earlier, NHS England also specifies the form and content of accounting information that CCGs must provide and a timetable for submission.

CCG budgets include a maximum allowance to cover administration or running costs. Although they can choose to undertake some or all of these roles themselves, they have the flexibility to use the money to buy in the services needed from commissioning support units (hosted by NHS England) or the private sector. For 2013/14 this 'running cost allowance' has been set at a maximum of £25 per head of population.

At a more detailed level, NHS England has set out in its 2013/14 planning guidance[8] five key measures that it will use in relation to CCG financial accountability:

* financial forecast outturn and performance against plan
* an assessment of the range of risk inherent in plans and mitigation strategies
* underlying financial position after adjusting for non-recurrent items
* triangulation of spend and activity between commissioning and provider plans
* delivery of running cost targets.

Non-foundation NHS trusts

Non-foundation NHS trusts have a number of statutory financial duties – i.e. duties that are a formal requirement as laid down in statute through Parliament. The principal duty is to achieve a break-even position on revenue and expenditure taking one year with another. Trusts must also pay public dividend capital (PDC)[9] dividends and remain within a borrowing limit set by the Secretary of State.[10]

The requirement to break-even is set out in paragraph 2 of Schedule 5 of the *National Health Service Act 2006* and means that a trust must ensure that its revenue is not less than sufficient, taking one financial year with another, to meet outgoings properly charged to the statement of comprehensive income (SOCI). 'Taking one financial year with another' has been interpreted to mean that over a three or five year period, trusts are required to achieve a break-even position on their SOCI. This is to allow some flexibility where exceptional costs are incurred and when managing the financial recovery of a trust with serious financial difficulties.

There is also an annual break-even requirement that is sometimes referred to as an 'administrative duty'. This is monitored by the NHS Trust Development Authority (NHS TDA). An administrative duty is not the same as a statutory duty – rather it is an additional rule and regulation that clarifies or specifies how a trust will operate. Trusts must report on the achievement of their financial duties in the annual report and accounts.

Other administrative duties (each explained below) are to:

* manage within a pre-set external financing limit (EFL)
* meet the capital resource limit (CRL)
* comply with the *Better Payment Practice Code* for the payment of invoices.

---

[8] *Everyone Counts: Planning for Patients 2013/14*, NHS England, 2012.
[9] PDC is a form of long-term government finance on which trusts pay dividends to the Treasury.
[10] See paragraph 1(6) of Schedule 5 of the *NHS Act 2006*.

Non-foundation NHS Trust Administrative Duties

External financing limit

The EFL was established to control the amount a trust could spend on capital in a year and included all sources of finance (internal, external or from the Department of Health). However, over time the EFL came to be seen as a 'financing limit' – i.e. the maximum amount that a trust could draw from the Department over and above what it could generate from its own operations. Since 2008/09, the EFL has been set to include cash provided for capital purposes from:

* the Department (PDC and loans)
* internal generation
* external sources.

The EFL is an absolute financial duty. There is no tolerance above the EFL target as it is designed to control the cash expenditure of the NHS as a whole to the level agreed by Parliament.

The EFL sets a limit on the level of cash that an NHS trust may:

* draw from either external sources or its own cash reserves (a positive EFL) **OR**
* repay to external sources for capital borrowing (a negative EFL).

A target EFL is set at the start of the financial year by the Department of Health and the trust is expected to manage its resources to ensure it achieves the target – it must not overshoot the EFL as it is a departmental duty.

Capital resource limit

NHS trusts must control capital expenditure to meet their CRL. The CRL is set by the Department of Health and is the total of the following:

* depreciation
* revenue surpluses
* proceeds from asset sales
* capital loans
* funding from central funds (provided as PDC).

Better Payment Practice Code

NHS trusts must comply with the *Better Payment Practice Code*. A target (currently 95%) is set at the start of each year by the Department of Health for the value and volume of invoices that must be paid within 30 days of receipt.

NHS foundation trusts

FTs' financial targets differ from NHS trusts. There is no requirement for FTs to break-even, remain within an EFL or remain within a CRL. This reflects the different financial regime that FTs operate within. Although FTs are allowed to incur deficits and operate on a similar basis to commercial organisations, they must operate effectively, efficiently and economically so that they remain going concerns. In effect this means that FTs' main financial target is to remain solvent. As part of the NHS, FTs are also required to demonstrate high standards of financial stewardship in relation to their use of public funds.

Monitor sets the financial framework within which FTs operate and gives each FT a financial risk rating of 1 (high risk) to 5 (low risk). The financial risk rating system is set out in the *Compliance Framework* which is updated annually. From mid-way through 2013/14, the *Compliance Framework* will be replaced by the *Risk Assessment Framework* (the two sets of guidance are running in parallel for the first six months of 2013/14).

Financial Performance Management

The Department of Health requires the financial performance of NHS bodies to be monitored on a regular basis. The first element of the financial performance management process is the financial plan. All NHS organisations are required to undertake medium term financial planning and as part of this process, the organisation must plan to achieve its financial duties. The plan must cover all expected sources of revenue and expenditure and the full range of responsibilities under the management of the organisation.

NHS organisations must then report regularly on their financial performance against the plan submitted at the start of the financial year to ensure that there is effective financial management of NHS resources. This information is collated by NHS England (for CCGs) and the NHS Trust Development Authority (NHS TDA) (for non-foundation NHS trusts) and reported to the Department of Health. The timing of the reporting to the Department is designed to reflect the information requirements of Parliament which are:

- reporting the national revenue and capital financial position
- to inform Parliamentary estimates
- to ensure effective management of the Department of Health 'vote' (i.e. the money allocated to the Department by the Treasury).

Chief finance officers are expected to inform NHS England/NHS TDA if there are any significant variances against plans and to ensure that appropriate recovery plans are put into place. At present this is achieved by completion of in-year financial monitoring and accounts (FMA) forms and associated commentary.

Although Monitor does not performance manage FTs in the same way, it does receive information from them on a regular basis with the frequency depending on each FT's risk rating. Monitor compares the information received against the annual plan submitted at the beginning of the year and takes action if there are significant deviations.

Non-financial Performance Standards and Targets

As well as financial duties, there are a number of other targets that NHS bodies are required to meet. The *Health and Social Care (Community Health and Standards) Act 2003* established the power for the Secretary of State for Health to set standards which are published by the Department of Health. Guidance issued by the National Institute for Health and Care Excellence (NICE) is also an important element of the standards system.

From 2008/09 to 2012/13, the Department of Health set out in its *Operating Frameworks* health and service priorities for the year ahead. From 2013/14, this role was assumed by NHS England which issued *Everyone Counts: Planning for Patients 2013/14* in December 2012. This identifies a number of indicators and milestones that are used to assess how well NHS bodies are delivering their plans, grouped under four key areas:

• listening to patients
• focusing on outcomes
• rewarding excellence
• improving knowledge and data.

As part of the focus on outcomes, providers are required to publish consultant level data about survival rates and quality of care for ten specialties including cardio vascular and orthopaedic surgery. From 2014/15 publication of this information will be a contractual obligation.

Performance Assessment

The Department of Health

The Department of Health introduced *The Performance Framework* in 2009 to assess non-foundation provider organisations against minimum standards. In April 2012, it was revised and now applies to all NHS providers that are not yet FTs.

The approach involves assessing performance across two domains – finance and quality of service and for each there are a series of indicators, performance thresholds and a scoring system. For quality of service, performance is measured across three areas – integrated performance measures; user experience and CQC registration status.

The results of the assessment are published each quarter in the Department of Health's *The Quarter* publication. Based on the scores achieved, organisations are categorised as either:

• performing
• performance under review
• underperforming.

The results from the performance framework are published alongside overall 'Tripartite Formal Agreement' (TFA)[11] red, amber, green (RAG) ratings.

---

[11] A TFA sets out the commitments made by a trust, the NHS TDA and the Department of Health that will enable achievement of FT status.

External audit

The public is entitled to expect that money raised by local or national taxation is properly accounted for. To provide an assurance that this is the case, there is a need (among other things) for a wide-ranging and independent external audit covering both the financial statements and the organisation's arrangements for securing value for money from its use of resources.

At present, for all non-foundation NHS trusts and CCGs the financial audit regime is the responsibility of the Audit Commission. This will continue until the Commission is abolished – its last year of operation is expected to be 2014/15. The Commission's responsibilities involve:

- appointing external auditors who audit a body's annual financial statements
- setting the required standards of appointed auditors
- regulating the quality of audits.

External auditors must follow the Audit Commission's *Code of Audit Practice* which requires them to review and report on:

- the annual accounts
- arrangements for securing economy, efficiency and effectiveness in the use of resources.

By exception, auditors must also report when the annual governance statement does not comply with Department of Health requirements.

The *Audit Commission Act 1998* also provides auditors with the power to report where they have specific concerns arising from their audits of NHS organisations – see chapter 12 for more details.

The external auditor is required to issue an annual audit letter to Board members at the conclusion of each year's audit. The letter acts as a brief for the Board and summarises the major issues arising from the audit which the auditor wishes to raise.

All FTs must have their accounts audited by independent external auditors who are appointed by the FT's Council of Governors. Monitor's *Audit Code for NHS Foundation Trusts* prescribes the way in which an FT's external auditors must carry out their functions. The role and the reporting duties of FTs' auditors are very similar to those of Audit Commission appointed auditors. Whilst Monitor does not appoint auditors, it does have a role in assessing the quality of audits.

Internal audit

Internal audit is defined in the *UK Public Sector Internal Audit Standards* as 'an independent, objective assurance and consulting activity designed to add value and improve an organisation's operations. It helps an organisation accomplish its objectives by bringing a systematic, disciplined approach to evaluate and improve the effectiveness of risk management, control and governance processes'. These standards apply to all NHS organisations from April 2013.

All NHS bodies (including CCGs and FTs) are required to have an internal audit function and the Head of Internal Audit's annual opinion is used by the Accountable/Accounting Officer to inform the annual governance statement.

As the definition above indicates, the internal audit service fulfils two functions – assurance and consultancy. The first involves providing an independent and objective opinion to the Accountable/Accounting Officer, Board and audit committee on the extent to which risk management, control and governance arrangements support the aims of the organisation. In this context, risk management, control and governance means the policies, procedures and operations established to ensure:

- the achievement of objectives
- the appropriate assessment of risk
- the reliability of internal and external reporting and accountability processes
- compliance with applicable laws and regulations
- compliance with the behavioural and ethical standards set for the organisation.

The second involves providing an independent and objective consultancy service specifically to help line management improve the organisation's risk management, control and governance. When performing consultancy services, the internal auditor must maintain objectivity and not take on management responsibility.

Internal Reporting

For organisations to run effectively, the governing body and managers at all levels need to receive up to date financial and non-financial performance information on a timely basis. This information needs to be derived from the same financial system that is used for external reporting purposes – this ensures consistency in reports and that decisions throughout the organisation are made on the same basis.

Reporting to governing bodies

NHS governing bodies (or Boards) are responsible for ensuring that there are high standards of financial stewardship through effective financial planning, financial control and ensuring value for money. To achieve this, NHS Boards require an effective system of financial and performance reporting that is accurate and timely so that they can take early and corrective action where necessary. It is for the governing body to decide the form and content of the reports it requires and it should review its information needs regularly. The Board should also make use of assessments carried out by external bodies.

> **Examples of Financial Information that is reported to Boards each month**
>
> - Performance against the achievement of statutory and departmental duties and targets
> - In-year revenue and expenditure position and year-end forecasts, including an analysis of financial risks, the likelihood of them arising and how they will be managed
> - Activity levels linked to financial data
> - Progress on the achievement of any cost improvement programmes and financial recovery plans

- Statement of financial position
- Cash forecast
- Aged receivable and payable balances including actions taken and progress made
- Losses
- Performance of outsourced services
- Progress against internal and external audit recommendations
- Progress on major capital schemes
- Staffing and establishment reports

As well as considering monthly reports, there is some financial information that the Board needs to consider every year, including:

- the annual accounts
- financial plans
- the annual audit letter which summarises the key issues identified during the external audit.

The Board should also be updated and advised regularly on the nature and development of new systems and initiatives in the NHS so that it is better able to understand the implications and prepared to manage the impact when implementation takes place.

Reporting to budget holders

The reporting of performance against the budget and any corrective action taken as a result is an essential element of financial management in the NHS. Reporting to budget holders must therefore be sufficiently detailed to ensure that all significant variances are identified and issues that need to be corrected are highlighted.

Budget monitoring information is produced at a range of levels, allowing managers to see not only summary performance, but also the performance of individual departments and teams. The exact nature of this reporting depends on the organisation's management structure but in each case it is essential that the information is timely, accurate and fit for purpose. To ensure accuracy, financial commitments should be recognised as soon as possible and reflected in the monthly financial reports. Without accurate budget reporting at budget holder level, costs cannot be controlled properly. These reports are often referred to as the 'management accounts'. Chapter 14 looks in more detail at revenue planning and budgeting.

Over recent years a development in the management accounting field has introduced the concepts of service line reporting (SLR) and patient level costing. A service line is a distinct clinical operating unit, with clearly definable activity, income and costs. SLR is made possible through the payment by results (PbR) system and allows a trust to see the profitability of each of its service lines, not just the overall position. This approach allows clinicians and managers to better understand cost drivers (i.e. the factors that lead to costs being incurred) and the financial effect of clinical decisions. It also provides the evidence to support strategic decisions such as investment and expansion of particular service lines.

Patient level costing is the natural extension of service line reporting. Whereas SLR analyses activity, income and costs at departmental level, patient level costing assigns income and costs to individual patient activity (for example, a 'patient spell',[12] outpatient attendance or diagnostic test). This is more complex and requires detailed recording of all activity relating to a patient spell – for example, operating theatre time; the time spent by individual clinicians and the amount of drugs and other medical supplies used. However, the benefit is increased accuracy both in terms of reporting and in relation to reference cost returns, on which the PbR tariff is based.

Chapter 17 looks more closely at costing and chapter 18 at PbR.

> **Key Learning Points**
> - All NHS bodies have a statutory duty to prepare an annual report and accounts that is audited
> - The annual accounts must be prepared in accordance with international financial reporting standards and additional guidance is provided in the form of manuals by the Department of Health/NHS England/Monitor
> - The annual governance statement forms part of the annual report and accounts and reflects on the arrangements that the NHS body has in place to manage and control risk
> - Quality accounts (or reports) must be prepared by bodies providing healthcare and focus on the quality of the care provided and areas for improvement in the future
> - CCGs must prepare an annual commissioning plan
> - The annual report is a review of the past year and performance against targets
> - All regulatory bodies undertake financial monitoring throughout the year and require financial information on a regular basis
> - All NHS bodies have financial targets which they must meet. Some are statutory and others are administrative
> - Additional assurance over the financial reporting of NHS bodies is provided by external auditors
> - All NHS bodies must have an internal audit service that fulfils two key functions – assurance and consultancy
> - NHS bodies are responsible for monitoring their own financial performance from the overall corporate level through to budget holders
> - Governing bodies should think carefully about their information needs to ensure that they can properly direct the organisation.

---

[12] A 'spell' covers all that happens to a patient from when he or she is admitted through to discharge.

References and Further Reading

Health and Social Care Act 2012: www.legislation.gov.uk/ukpga/2012/7/contents/enacted

NHS Act 2006: www.legislation.gov.uk/ukpga/2006/41/contents

International Accounting Standards Board: www.ifrs.org

Financial Reporting Manual, HM Treasury: www.hm-treasury.gov.uk/frem_index.htm

Manual for Accounts, Department of Health: www.info.doh.gov.uk/doh/finman.nsf

NHS Foundation Trust Annual Reporting Manual, Monitor:
www.monitor-nhsft.gov.uk/home/news-events-and-publications/our-publications/browse-category/guidance-foundation-trusts/mandat-5

Managing Public Money, HM Treasury: www.hm-treasury.gov.uk/psr_mpm_index.htm

National Health Service (Quality Accounts) Regulations 2010, National Health Service (Quality Accounts) Amendment Regulations 2011 www.legislation.gov.uk/uksi/2012/3081/contents/made

Changes to Quality Accounts reporting arrangements, Department of Health, 2013:
www.dh.gov.uk/health/2013/01/changes-qa-reporting/

NHS England Planning Guidance: Everyone Counts: Planning for Patients 2013/14:
www.england.nhs.uk/everyonecounts/

Compliance Framework, Monitor: www.monitor-nhsft.gov.uk/home/news-events-and-publications/our-publications/browse-category/guidance-foundation-trusts/mandat-4

Risk Assessment Framework, Monitor, 2013: www.monitor-nhsft.gov.uk/home/news-events-and-publications/latest-press-releases/monitor-consults-risk-assessment-framework

The Quarter, Department of Health:
https://www.gov.uk/government/publications/the-quarter-quarter-2-2012-13

Code of Audit Practice, Audit Commission:
www.audit-commission.gov.uk/audit-regime/codes-of-audit-practice/

Audit Code for NHS Foundation Trusts, Monitor: www.monitor-nhsft.gov.uk/home/our-publications/browse-category/guidance-foundation-trusts/mandatory-guidance/audit-code-nhs-f

UK Public Sector Internal Auditing Standards, 2012:
www.gov.uk/government/publications/uk-public-sector-internal-audit-standards-published

Chapter 12: How the NHS is Regulated

> ## Overview
>
> A key influence on the governance arrangements of all organisations is the external environment within which they operate and the statutory and regulatory requirements that they are expected to satisfy. Most NHS organisations are tightly constrained and so it is particularly important that they are aware of their operational context. They also need to have processes in place as part of their overall arrangements to enable them to monitor, respond and adhere to legislative and regulatory developments.
>
> Chapter 9 outlined the roles, responsibilities and accountabilities of the key sector-wide regulators that affect the NHS (Monitor, the Care Quality Commission and the National Institute for Health and Care Excellence). This chapter focuses on the approach of those regulators and inspection agencies that have a direct impact on NHS organisations in terms of their finance and governance arrangements.

The Role of Government

Given that it is a top political priority, it is no surprise that the Government devotes considerable time and effort to ensuring that the NHS operates in an accountable and open way and that it achieves agreed objectives and targets. It is also important to remember that all NHS bodies are creatures of statute – they must always act within the law and never beyond their legal powers. All their powers come from Parliament, through Acts and statutory instruments.

The Secretary of State has a direct influence on the governance arrangements of NHS bodies and on their powers and activities – the only exception at present (2013/14) is that for NHS foundation trusts (FTs) governance arrangements are set by Monitor.

The most obvious area where the Secretary of State has an impact is in relation to the overall structure of the health service.

At a more detailed level, the Secretary of State sets down the statutory powers, structures and reporting lines for different types of organisation. Requirements and duties that NHS organisations must follow are set out in primary and secondary legislation and in circulars, directions and guidelines – these are issued via the Department of Health and NHS England.

The Role of Regulatory, Inspection and Audit Agencies

NHS organisations are subject to regulation and inspection from a wide range of bodies that are independent of Government and the NHS. These include national agencies and specific organisations linked to the many different professions involved in the delivery of healthcare –

ranging from the Royal Colleges[1] to the Care Quality Commission, the General Medical Council to HM Revenue and Customs.

In an environment where demonstrating high quality performance and the effective use of public funds is essential, the role of regulatory and inspection agencies and their impact on an organisation's reputation and morale cannot be underestimated. It is therefore critical that NHS bodies are aware of the approach and requirements of each organisation and that appropriate mechanisms are in place to facilitate the inspection process and respond to any recommendations or advice that are issued, to the organisation itself or to the wider NHS.

Audit Commission

The Government is in the process of abolishing the Audit Commission which was established in 1983 and is now a non-departmental public body sponsored by the Department for Communities and Local Government. The intention as set out in a 'key milestones table' published alongside the *Draft Local Audit Bill* is that the Commission's last year of operation will be 2014/15. Until then it remains responsible for ensuring that public money is spent economically, efficiently and effectively to achieve high quality public services and better outcomes for everyone. In particular, the Commission is responsible for the financial audit regime for all non-foundation NHS trusts and clinical commissioning groups (CCGs). This entails:

- appointing external auditors who audit a body's annual financial statements
- setting the required standards of appointed auditors
- regulating the quality of audits.

External auditors must follow the Audit Commission's *Code of Audit Practice* which requires them to review and report on:

- the annual accounts
- arrangements for securing economy, efficiency and effectiveness in the use of resources.

By exception, auditors must also report when the annual governance statement does not comply with Department of Health requirements – see chapter 11 for more details about NHS accounts.

The *Audit Commission Act 1998* provides auditors with the power to report where they have specific concerns arising from their audits of NHS organisations via:

- public interest reports – section 8 of the Act requires auditors to consider whether to issue a report in the public interest on any significant matter coming to their notice

---

[1] 'Royal Colleges' refers to a range of representative organisations for different medical specialists such as GPs, surgeons, anaesthetists, radiologists etc. Details can be found on the Academy of Medical Royal Colleges website: www.aomrc.org.uk/.

- reference to the Secretary of State – section 19 requires the auditor to refer matters to the Secretary of State for Health if he or she has reason to believe that an NHS organisation has made a decision that involves, or may involve, unlawful expenditure.

The external auditor is required to issue an annual audit letter to the NHS body's Board members at the conclusion of each year's audit. The letter acts as a brief for the Board and summarises the major issues arising from the audit which the auditor wishes to raise.

The Audit Commission does not have a role in relation to FTs.

National Audit Office (NAO)

The National Audit Office (NAO) reports to Parliament on the spending of central government money. To be able to do this the NAO:

- conducts financial audits of all government departments and agencies and many other public bodies – this includes the Department of Health and its arms' length bodies (for example, Monitor and the CQC)
- reports to Parliament on the value for money that public bodies achieve with the public money they receive.

For the NHS this means that, as well as auditing the Department of Health's annual resource account, the NAO audits the annual accounts of each of the Department's arms' length bodies, the summarised accounts of NHS trusts and the consolidated accounts of FTs. The NAO is therefore responsible for the audit of NHS England (including the consolidation of CCG accounts into NHS England's account) but **not** for the audit of CCGs themselves (they fall under the Audit Commission's regime until it is abolished).

When carrying out its auditing functions, the NAO places reliance on and takes assurance from the work carried out by external auditors on the underlying accounts of individual NHS bodies.

The NAO's value for money activities in the NHS are designed to provides assurance to Parliament on 'the extent to which the NHS and the Department of Health deliver economically, efficiently and effectively across the health care sector'.[2]

The Government's intention is that the NAO will take over responsibility for determining and maintaining the *Code of Audit Practice* once the Audit Commission is abolished.

Care Quality Commission

As we saw in chapter 9, the Care Quality Commission (CQC) was established to regulate 'essential standards of quality and safety', which are set out in the *Health and Social Care Act 2008*. The Commission's remit covers:

---

[2] NAO website.

- NHS providers
- adult social care providers
- independent healthcare providers
- dentists
- private ambulances
- NHS out-of-hours services (that are not GP practices)
- GPs and NHS walk-in centres (that do not provide out of hours services).

Regulatory approach – registration and compliance system

The CQC regulates through a registration and compliance system, where registration represents a licence to operate. Once registered to carry out regulated activities a provider must show that it is meeting the essential standards of quality and safety. In order to be licensed by Monitor, a provider must first be registered with the CQC.

In April 2014, CQC and Monitor plan to implement a joint licence for all NHS providers who are regulated by both organisations.

CQC monitors a provider's compliance with essential standards using a system of information management and analysis, which informs inspection visits to registered services. The CQC uses and checks many different types of information about providers, including clinical performance data and information from people who use services, public representative groups, and other organisations and regulators, such as Monitor.

Essential standards of quality and safety

As mentioned above, the essential standards are set out in regulations issued under the *Health and Social Care Act 2008*.[3] These regulations describe 28 essential standards of quality and safety that people who use health and adult social care services should expect.

The CQC looks at all 28 essential standards when monitoring the compliance of providers, but its judgement framework has a particular focus on the 16 essential standards and associated outcomes that most directly relate to the quality and safety of care experienced by people using a service.

The 16 Essential CQC Standards

1. Care and welfare of people who use services
2. Assessing and monitoring the quality of service provision
3. Safeguarding vulnerable people who use services
4. Cleanliness and infection control
5. Management of medicines
6. Meeting nutritional needs

---

[3] Specifically, the *Health and Social Care Act 2008 (Regulated Activities) Regulations 2010*, and the *Care Quality Commission (Registration) Regulations 2009*.

7. Safety and suitability of premises
8. Safety, availability and suitability of equipment
9. Respecting and involving people who use services
10. Consent to care and treatment
11. Complaints management
12. Records management
13. Requirements relating to workers
14. Staffing
15. Supporting workers
16. Co-operating with other providers.

Conditions of registration

When providers first register with the CQC they might have compliance conditions attached to their registration where the CQC has identified concerns about non-compliance. In such instances, providers must implement an agreed time-bound improvement plan for the conditions to be removed or the CQC will take enforcement action.

In addition, the CQC can apply 'routine restrictive conditions' to providers as part of their registration. These conditions will place a limit or a restriction on what activity can be carried out. It may be linked to a location, regulated activity, service type, or specific activity. An example of a routine restrictive condition is defining a location where a regulated activity can be carried out or the need for a registered manager. If changes occur to a service that impact on the routine restrictive conditions, the provider must inform the CQC and apply for a variation to their registration or face enforcement action.

See chapter 9 for more about the CQC's status and role and the CQC website for further information on its regulatory activities.

CQC response to the Mid Staffordshire NHS Foundation Trust Public Inquiry Report (the Francis Inquiry)

The CQC's inspection regime has always focussed on ensuring that health and social care services provide people with safe, high quality care that meets the fundamental standards set out above. However, in response to the recommendations set out in the Francis Inquiry, the CQC's inspections of acute and mental health hospitals have a particular focus on:

- safety
- caring
- effectiveness
- how well the hospital is led.

The CQC is also appointing a Chief Inspector of Hospitals and introducing expert inspection teams at both the local and national level (the latter to carry out in depth reviews of hospitals with significant or long standing problems). At the same time, the Commission intends to:

- identify, predict and respond more quickly to varying standards of care by using data, intelligence and evidence in a more sophisticated way
- 'listen better to people's experience of moving between different services, work better with other regulators and partners to share information and evidence and coordinate our inspections and activities and publish better information for the public, including an overall rating of a service'.[4]

Monitor

As we saw in chapter 9, Monitor is an independent corporate body established under the *Health and Social Care (Community Health and Standards) Act 2003*. At present, it is responsible for licensing, monitoring and regulating FTs and assesses risk and intervenes to ensure compliance with all aspects of the licence.[5] It will continue to fulfil this role until 2016 but (since April 2013) has assumed a wider role as 'sector regulator for health' – this involves licensing all providers of NHS funded healthcare (FTs from April 2013 and all other providers from April 2014).

Regulatory approach – the compliance/risk assessment framework

Monitor has established a risk-based approach to regulation which means that assessments of risk are used to determine the level and depth of monitoring that an FT is subject to. The approach was originally set out in Monitor's *Compliance Framework* which it reviewed (and consulted on) each year. During 2013/14 this will be replaced with a *Risk Assessment Framework* that focuses more on the continuity of key services and an organisation's ability to provide them.[6] Where possible incidents of failures and breaches that arise under the *Compliance Framework* will be carried forward for oversight under the *Risk Assessment Framework*.

Under both frameworks, Monitor focuses on two risk areas – finance and governance – and its assessment relies primarily on the information it receives directly from FTs (including annual plans and in-year monitoring submissions). Monitor also considers third party reports on a variety of specific issues, in particular those of other regulatory bodies.

Finance risk rating

Under the *Compliance Framework*, a 'financial scorecard' is used to generate a finance risk rating (FRR) and this is split into four criteria. For each criterion a score of 1 to 5 is awarded with 1 indicating a high risk of breaching licence conditions and 5 a low risk with no financial regulatory concerns.

---

[4] CQC press release on the Francis Inquiry, 26/01/13.
[5] An FT's licence sets out the basis for its establishment and future operation.
[6] The compliance and risk assessment frameworks run alongside each other for the first six months of 2013/14.

> **Compliance Framework – the four areas looked at for the Financial Scorecard**
> - Achievement of plan
> - Underlying performance
> - Financial efficiency
> - Liquidity

As mentioned, one purpose of the FRR is to assist Monitor in determining the frequency with which it needs to monitor the organisation or intervene as appropriate. Another is to grant autonomy to high performing organisations in order that they may maximise the financial freedoms (including borrowing) and responsibilities available to FTs while at the same time ensuring proper risk management. For example, FTs set their own level of capital expenditure and in so doing must decide on the best method of financing such expenditure.

Continuity of services risk rating

Under the *Risk Assessment Framework* (that applies from mid-2013/14 onwards), the number of metrics reduce to two – each with an equal weighting:

- liquidity
- capital service capacity.

These metrics are designed to identify the risk to the continued provision of commissioner requested services;[7] give an indication of the ability to meet both operating and financing cash demands and ultimately whether a provider is likely to continue as a going concern.

Governance risk rating

Under the *Compliance Framework*, the governance risk rating focuses on the degree to which FTs are complying with the governance conditions of the licence and looks at five criteria.

> **Governance Risk Rating under the Compliance Framework – the Five Criteria**
> 1. Performance against service measures
> 2. Third party views in relation to the Care Quality Commission (CQC) and the NHS Litigation Authority (NHSLA)
> 3. Delivery of commissioner requested services
> 4. Other Board statement failures where Boards have failed to accurately self-certify and the failure is material
> 5. Other factors (which can include failure to meet the statutory requirements of other bodies).

---

[7] These are services that will be considered by the commissioner for protection should the provider fail.

Under the *Risk Assessment Framework* (i.e. from mid-2013/14 onwards), this will be replaced by:

- a single corporate governance statement confirming compliance at the statement date and anticipated compliance for the next financial year
- a governance rating covering six categories:
  1. CQC judgements
  2. service performance against national access standards
  3. performance against selected elements of the *NHS Outcomes Framework*
  4. relevant information from third parties for example, an ad hoc report from HealthWatch England
  5. quality governance metrics including staff and patient information in relation to the quality of care provided
  6. the risk to the continuity of services (the so-called 'continuity of services regime')
- forward plans which may trigger governance concerns
- periodic external governance reviews.

How FTs work with Monitor

The relationship between FTs and Monitor is based on effective self-governance and self-certification of compliance, with the FT's Board of Directors taking primary responsibility for compliance with the licence. The Chairperson has a key role in ensuring that the Board of Directors monitors the performance of the FT in an effective way and satisfies itself that effective action is taken to remedy problems as they arise.

FTs must initially report to Monitor annually (by way of an annual plan) and on a quarterly basis to ensure that they comply with their licence.

Where FTs are experiencing significant financial, service or governance problems, oversight is more intensive and monthly reporting may be required; the intensity of monitoring will be guided by risk assessments.

Monitor's intervention and enforcement powers

Under the *Health and Social Care Act 2012*, Monitor has extensive powers to intervene in the event that a licensed provider is failing to comply with its licence conditions.

Monitor's Intervention Powers under the Health and Social Care Act 2012

Section 89 enables Monitor to revoke a provider's licence.

Section 105 of the Act gives Monitor power to require a provider to take specific or a 'discretionary requirement'. This may take the form of:

- a compliance requirement: an instruction from Monitor to take specific steps
- a restoration requirement: requiring the provider to restore the situation to the position before the breach

---

- a variable monetary penalty – likely if there is significant potential for the breach to reoccur.

Section 106 of the Act enables Monitor to accept a commitment from a provider to take steps to ensure that a breach of the licence condition does not continue or reoccur – an 'enforcement undertaking'. Acceptance is at Monitor's discretion and will depend on individual circumstances.

Section 111 gives Monitor power to impose additional licence conditions and remove, suspend or disqualify director(s) and/or governor(s).

Using 'specific enforcement powers' granted under sections 105 and 106 of the Act, Monitor can also take action against those healthcare bodies failing to provide information as required in its role as sector regulator including NHS England and CCGs. As sector regulator, Monitor also has powers concurrent with the Office of Fair Trading to apply competition law in the healthcare sector.

In addition, Monitor has a duty to 'prevent providers from taking actions that could undermine their continued ability to deliver services' (the 'continuity of service regime'). This can involve Monitor in helping providers who are having problems (for example, by requiring them to appoint turnaround experts to help avoid failure) or (in exceptional circumstances) appointing a 'trust special administrator' to take control of the provider's business and work with commissioners to make sure that patients can still access services. Where a provider is in financial difficulty, Monitor has a duty to make available a source of finance to cover the costs of administration, via a risk pool arrangement – a fund that is built up via levies on providers and commissioners.

In the future, there will be a significant emphasis on provider self-awareness and self-monitoring – in other words, licensed providers must be aware of any actions they take which may cause a breach in licence conditions. Monitor plans to adopt a proportionate approach whereby action can be informal or formal and relative to the steps taken by the provider concerned to resolve the issues itself.

Monitor has recognised the importance of effective governance in the success of every FT and has published a *Code of Governance for NHS Foundation Trusts* to promote key principles and how they should be applied in practice. The document is based closely on the *UK Corporate Governance Code*, which is the nearest equivalent from the private sector.

NHS Trust Development Authority (NHS TDA)

As we saw in chapter 3, the NHS TDA is responsible for overseeing all remaining NHS trusts and for supporting them as they move towards foundation status. It has issued detailed planning guidance[8] that sets out what non-foundation trusts are expected to deliver during 2013/14 and also how their progress will be monitored.

---

[8] *Toward High Quality Sustainable Services: Planning Guidance for NHS Trust Boards for 2013/14*, NHS TDA, 2013.

The key document that the NHS TDA uses to monitor performance is the 'integrated plan' which each trust must prepare by 31st March. This plan is designed to show how the trust will:

- deliver high quality, sustainable services for the patients and community it serves
- meet the expectations, priorities and measures set out in the *NHS Constitution, NHS Mandate* and *NHS Outcomes Framework*
- continue to move towards achieving FT status in line with the trajectories set out in its Tripartite Formal Agreement (TFA).[9]

Each plan must be signed off by the NHS TDA – if there are any concerns about its deliverability or credibility sign-off does not take place and further discussions are held.

The NHS TDA's planning guidance identifies four other 'core elements' to their approach that will affect trusts as they work towards FT status.

The Four Core Elements of the NHS TDA's Approach

1. Oversight – a consistent approach to the way trusts are monitored in relation to quality, finance, key deliverables (including progress against plans) and progress towards becoming an FT
2. Escalation – clear rules that the NHS TDA will use to decide when a trust 'needs additional support, further direction or even, in extreme cases, intervention if it is not able to achieve its goals'
3. Development – support via the NHS TDA's local teams and work with other national bodies such as the NHS Leadership Academy
4. Approvals – a streamlined approach to assessing FT applications, proposed transactions and capital projects.

See the NHS TDA's website for further guidance.

NHS England

NHS England is responsible for authorising CCGs and holding them to account both for improving outcomes to patients and for getting the best possible value from the money they are allocated.

NHS England has issued detailed planning guidelines[10] that set out what CCGs are expected to deliver during 2013/14 and also how their progress will be monitored. The key document for every CCG is its annual operating plan which must show that it can deliver the *NHS Mandate* and improve patient outcomes within the resources allocated to it.

---

[9] A TFA sets out the commitments made by a trust, the NHS TDA and the Department of Health that will enable achievement of FT status.
[10] *Everyone Counts: Planning for Patients 2013/14*, NHS England, 2012.

NHS England has a statutory duty to carry out an annual assessment of each CCG that focuses on CCGs' own statutory duties to:

- improve the quality of services
- reduce inequalities
- obtain appropriate professional advice
- ensure public involvement
- meet financial duties
- take account of the local Joint Health and Wellbeing Strategy.

The planning guidelines make clear that the assessment approach is based on the six domains used for CCG authorisation and that 'as the oversight body charged with assessing clinical commissioning groups against their statutory duties, NHS England will provide a single consistent approach to each of these areas.'

CCG Authorisation – the Six Domains

1. A strong clinical and multi-professional focus which brings real added value.
2. Meaningful engagement with patients, carers and their communities.
3. Clear and credible plans which continue to deliver the QIPP (quality, innovation, productivity and prevention) challenge within financial resources, in line with national requirements (including outcomes) and local joint health and wellbeing strategies.
4. Proper constitutional and governance arrangements, with the capacity and capability to deliver all their duties and responsibilities, including financial control, as well as effectively commission all the services for which they are responsible.
5. Collaborative arrangements for commissioning with other CCGs, local authorities and NHS England as well as the appropriate external commissioning support.
6. Great leaders who individually and collectively can make a real difference.

NHS England is also developing an 'assurance framework' in discussion with CCGs and other stakeholders that will 'identify how well CCGs are performing against their plans to improve services and deliver better outcomes for patients'.[11] The definitive version of this framework is due to be published in autumn 2013. See NHS England's website for details.

If a CCG is unable to fulfil its duties effectively or there is a significant risk of failure, NHS England has powers to intervene. These powers range from telling a CCG how it should discharge its functions through to dissolving a CCG completely if it is failing.

See chapters 4 and 5 for more about NHS England and CCGs.

Local Authorities

Since January 2003, local authorities with social services responsibilities have been able to establish committees of councillors to provide overview and scrutiny of local NHS bodies by virtue of powers set out in section 38 of the *Local Government Act 2000*. The ultimate aim is to

---

[11] *Interim CCG Assurance Framework 2013/14*, NHS England, 2013.

secure health improvement for local communities by encouraging authorities to look beyond their own service responsibilities to issues of wider concern to local people. This is achieved by giving democratically elected representatives the right to scrutinise how local health services are provided and developed for their constituents. This scrutiny role is extended by the 2012 Act to cover any provider of NHS funded services. Local authorities also now play a key role in public health and health improvement – see chapter 8 for details.

Other External Bodies

There is a wide range of other organisations with an interest in health which can affect governance arrangements. These include:

- professional bodies on both the clinical and managerial side. These organisations often have their own codes of conduct and disciplinary regimes that apply to their members. For example, the Royal Colleges and other independent audit and assurance bodies that provide an assurance to NHS organisations
- other government departments and agencies – for example, the Department for Communities and Local Government
- non-departmental public bodies, independent and local organisations (for example, local HealthWatch)
- representative bodies – for example, the British Medical Association (BMA), the NHS Confederation and UNISON
- think tanks and research organisations – such as the King's Fund
- the public – NHS organisations are required to engage with the public and conduct meaningful consultations.

Key Learning Points

- Government sets the overall structure for the NHS and all NHS bodies are creatures of statute
- NHS organisations must be aware of the approach and requirements of all relevant regulatory and inspection agencies
- Until it is abolished, the Audit Commission is responsible for ensuring that public money is spent efficiently, effectively and economically. It also appoints external auditors for non-foundation NHS trusts and CCGs
- The NAO conducts financial audits of all government departments including the Department of Health and its ALBs
- The CQC regulates providers of healthcare services via a system of registration and compliance with essential standards of quality and safety
- Monitor uses a risk based approach to regulation for FTs that focuses on finance and governance
- Monitor is also the sector regulator for health and has extensive powers to intervene if a licensed provider is not complying with its licence conditions
- The NHS TDA oversees and supports trusts moving towards foundation status – this role includes monitoring progress against integrated plans
- NHS England authorises and monitors CCGs and holds them to account
- Local authorities have a scrutiny role that extends to all providers of NHS funded services.

References and Further Reading

Academy of Medical Royal Colleges website: www.aomrc.org.uk/

Audit Commission: www.audit-commission.gov.uk/

Draft Local Audit Bill: www.parliament.uk/business/committees/committees-a-z/commons-select/draft-local-audit-bill-ad-hoc-committee/

Codes of Audit Practice, Audit Commission: www.audit-commission.gov.uk/audit-regime/codes-of-audit-practice/

Audit Commission Act 1998: www.legislation.gov.uk/ukpga/1998/18/contents

NAO: www.nao.org.uk

CQC: www.cqc.org.uk

Health and Social Care Act 2008: www.legislation.gov.uk/ukpga/2008/14/contents

Mid Staffordshire NHS Foundation Trust Public Inquiry Report (the Francis Inquiry), 2013: www.midstaffspublicinquiry.com/

CQC response to the Francis Report: www.cqc.org.uk/media/cqc-highlights-changes-following-francis-report

Monitor (including details of the Compliance and Risk Assessment Frameworks and the Code of Governance): www.monitor-nhsft.gov.uk/

The NHS Outcomes Framework: https://www.gov.uk/government/publications/nhs-outcomes-framework-2013-to-2014

Health and Social Care Act 2012: www.legislation.gov.uk/ukpga/2012/7/contents/enacted

Health and Social Care (Community Health and Standards) Act 2003: www.legislation.gov.uk/ukpga/2003/43/contents

NHS Trust Development Authority: www.ntda.nhs.uk/

Toward High Quality Sustainable Services: Planning Guidance for NHS Trust Boards for 2013/14, and Technical Guidance for Operating Plans, NHS TDA, 2012: www.ntda.nhs.uk/2012/12/21/nhs-tda-publishes-planning-technical-guidance-for-201314/

The NHS Constitution: www.gov.uk/government/publications/the-nhs-constitution-for-england

The NHS Mandate: http://mandate.dh.gov.uk/2012/11/13/nhs-mandate-published/

NHS England: www.england.nhs.uk/

Everyone Counts: Planning for Patients 2013/14 and Supporting Planning 2013/14 for CCGs, NHS England, 2012: www.england.nhs.uk/everyonecounts/

CCG Assurance Framework, NHS England, 2013: www.england.nhs.uk/2013/05/07/interim-ccg-af/

Local authority overview and scrutiny:
www.dh.gov.uk/health/2012/12/health-scrutiny-response/

Chapter 13: Governance – how NHS Organisations are Structured and Run

> **Overview**
>
> This chapter's focus is governance – a subject that has received considerable attention over the years following spectacular failings across all sectors of the economy – recent examples include the 2008 banking crisis and Mid Staffordshire NHS Foundation Trust. These (and many other) crises have demonstrated just how important good governance is to the wellbeing of an organisation and made clear that it encompasses everything that an organisation does, not just its administrative and support functions. In the NHS this means that effective governance is as much of a concern to a nurse or consultant as it is to an accountant or manager: achieving high standards of governance depends on everyone.
>
> Governance is a huge subject in its own right so this chapter focuses on key aspects relating to NHS finance. If you want to know more about the issues covered and about other aspects of governance, the HFMA produces an *Introductory Guide to NHS Governance*.

What is Governance?

The terms 'governance' and 'corporate governance' are now interchangeable but it was the use of corporate governance as a phrase in the 1992 Cadbury Committee Report[1] that initiated widespread debate in this area. Corporate governance was defined in that report as 'the system by which companies are directed and controlled' and its focus was on how companies were run, structured, led and held to account. It was this report that identified the three fundamental principles of good governance as being openness, integrity and accountability.

What this means in practice is that, on the structural side, governance is concerned with the systems, processes and controls that are in place to provide a sound framework for clear and accountable decision-making. In terms of leadership, governance is to do with the responsibilities, behaviour and approach of governing body members and senior managers and with the organisation's underlying culture and values. And in terms of accountability, governance is concerned with how those running the organisation explain and justify their actions to their stakeholders and how performance is managed.

Governance in the NHS

The NHS has been well aware of the importance of governance for many years with a wide range of separate regulatory frameworks and ethical codes in operation for the different professions working in NHS organisations. The challenge has been to bring together the practices and information systems of these different disciplines in such a way that they form an integrated and effective organisation-wide governance structure.

---

[1] *The Financial Aspects of Corporate Governance*, 1992.

The importance of having an integrated approach to governance (i.e. covering all aspects of governance including financial, clinical and organisational) along with high standards and an open culture has been heightened by failures which have dented public confidence in the NHS and raised questions over how NHS organisations are run. These have included:

- the Shipman crimes in 2003/04
- the Healthcare Commission's reports into Stoke Mandeville hospital (2006), Maidstone and Tunbridge Wells NHS Trust (2007) and Mid-Staffordshire NHS Foundation Trust (2009)
- the Francis Reports into Mid-Staffordshire NHS Foundation Trust (2010 and 2013).

In each case, clear linkages were drawn between the clinical scandals and the governance failings that allowed them to continue uncorrected. This has also driven home to governing bodies just how wide ranging their responsibilities and accountabilities are. In particular, they must assure themselves that the organisation:

- is providing high quality services in a safe environment – reflecting the fact that 'the primary purpose of the NHS, and everyone working within it, is to provide a high quality service, free at the point of delivery to everyone who needs it'[2]
- has staff that have been appropriately trained
- is engaging with stakeholders, most notably its patients
- is meeting its legal and regulatory requirements
- is meeting its strategic objectives.

Some of the more recent investigations into governance lapses have also underlined the need for an open and questioning culture and governance policies, procedures and structures that are comprehensive and work in practice, not just on paper.

Lessons from Governance Failings at Mid-Staffordshire NHS Foundation Trust

The Healthcare Commission's 2009 investigation into Mid-Staffordshire NHS Foundation Trust (where multiple management failures led to high mortality rates), found that the Trust, which was seeking to make financial savings in order to apply for foundation trust status, appeared to 'have lost sight of its real priorities'.

The 2010 report by Robert Francis QC revealed that deficiencies in staffing and governance extended over a period of more than 5 years and yet remained un-remedied by those responsible. His 2013 report went further and found that the trust had failed to listen to patients' concerns, correct deficiencies and tackle an 'insidious negative culture' that tolerated poor standards and clinical disengagement from managerial and leadership responsibilities. The report concluded that 'this failure was in part the consequence of allowing a focus on reaching national access targets, achieving financial balance and seeking foundation trust status at the cost of delivering acceptable standards of care.'

---

[2] *Quality Governance in the NHS - A guide for provider boards*, National Quality Board, 2011.

These (and other) incidents have emphasised just how important it is to see governance arrangements relating to clinical and quality spheres as an integral part of an organisation's overall approach, rather than the preserve of clinicians. The Quality Board's report made this clear when it stated that 'final and definitive responsibility for improvements, successful delivery, and equally failures, in the quality of care' lie with the provider organisation's Board and leaders. It goes on to say that as the 'primary focus of all NHS funded care is to be the delivering of improving quality and outcomes, the distinction between quality governance and clinical governance is less relevant as clinicians and managers are working towards the same ends – the delivery of the highest quality services.'

The Audit Commission's 2009 report *Taking it on Trust – a review of how NHS trusts and foundation trusts get their assurance* also emphasised the importance of an organisation-wide approach to governance when it suggested that future failures were likely unless a systematic approach is taken to identifying and managing key risks, and to evaluating assurances.

By now it should be clear why an effective and integrated approach to governance is so important and equally obvious that if an NHS organisation gets it wrong it can have a disastrous impact on patients and undermine public confidence in the service as a whole. But what does this mean NHS organisations need to do in practice?

In broad terms every organisation needs to focus on how they:

- are led and structured
- demonstrate that they are operating in line with the three fundamental governance principles – openness, integrity and accountability
- are meeting their statutory duties and strategic objectives
- ensure that they provide (or commission) high quality healthcare
- ensure that they operate economically, efficiently and effectively.

NHS bodies must also recognise that governance is as much about behaviour, values and attitudes as about structures, systems, processes and controls. There is no point having a comprehensive governance framework if no-one is committed to it or understands why it exists and what it is designed to achieve.

Elements of Governance

Effective governance arrangements should underpin all that an organisation does but it is helpful to break it down across three key elements – we will look at each in turn with a focus on financial aspects:

- culture and values (the people issues – for example, an organisation's leadership style and tone, openness and adherence to relevant legislation and codes of practice)
- structures and processes (for example, statutory and regulatory requirements, governing body/committee structures and internal policies and procedures)
- control frameworks (for example, financial controls, assurance, risk management, clinical audit, counter fraud and corruption).

Culture and Values

The *Good Governance Standard for Public Services* recognises that 'Good governance flows from a shared ethos or culture' and that it is 'the governing body that should take the lead in establishing and promoting values for the organisation and its staff'. In other words, the culture and values of an organisation are set from the top. In the context of the NHS this means that the behaviour, approach and leadership style of the governing body and senior management are critical in establishing an organisation's tone, 'feel' and direction.

This is re-iterated in the Professional Standards Authority for Health and Social Care's *Standards for Members of NHS Boards and Clinical Commissioning Group Governing Bodies in England* which sets out standards across three domains – personal behaviour; technical competence and business practices.

Leadership

Good leadership and management are crucial both to sound governance and to the overall vision and effectiveness of an organisation. Of particular relevance to the NHS is the NHS Leadership Academy's *Leadership Framework* developed in 2011. This framework sets out the expectations for leadership at every level of the system with four elements of leadership in each of seven domains. Each element has four stages of development – managing personal practice; leading a team; leading a service and leading a system.

Leadership Framework – the Seven Domains and Related 'Elements'

1. **Demonstrating personal qualities**: developing self-awareness; managing yourself; continuing personal development; acting with integrity
2. **Working with others**: developing networks; building and maintaining relationships; encouraging contribution; working within teams
3. **Managing services**: planning; managing resources; managing people; managing performance
4. **Improving services**: ensuring patient safety; critically evaluating; encouraging improvement and innovation; facilitating transformation
5. **Setting direction**: identifying the contexts for change; applying knowledge and evidence; making decisions; evaluating impact
6. **Creating the vision**: developing the vision of the organisation; influencing the vision of the wider healthcare system; communicating the vision; embodying the vision
7. **Delivering the strategy**: framing the strategy; developing the strategy; implementing the strategy; embedding the strategy.

Principles of public life

Everyone involved in the public sector brings their own personality, experience and behaviour with them. However, the public provides the resources for which they are responsible and, as a result, certain ethical standards and values are expected of them – these standards are known as the *Seven Principles of Public Life* and were set out by the Nolan Committee in 1995.

The Nolan Principles of Public Life

Selflessness – holders of public office should take decisions solely in terms of the public interest. They should not do so in order to gain financial or other material benefits for themselves, their family, or their friends.

Integrity – holders of public office should not place themselves under any financial or other obligation to outside individuals or organisations that might influence them in the performance of their official duties.

Objectivity – in carrying out public business, including making public appointments, awarding contracts, or recommending individuals for rewards and benefits, holders of public office should make choices on merit.

Accountability – holders of public office are accountable for their decisions and actions to the public and must submit to whatever scrutiny is appropriate to their office.

Openness – holders of public office should be as open as possible about all the decisions and actions that they take. They should give reasons for their decisions and restrict information only when the wider public interest clearly demands it.

Honesty – holders of public office have a duty to declare any private interests relating to their public duties and to take steps to resolve any conflicts arising in a way that protects the public interest.

Leadership – holders of public office should promote and support these principles by leadership and example.

The Treasury's guidance document, *Managing Public Money* also sets out the standards which it expects all public services to deliver which overlap with the Nolan principles:

Managing Public Money Standards	
Honesty	Transparency
Fairness	Accountability
Impartiality	Objectivity
Integrity	Accuracy
Openness	Reliability

The Treasury adds that organisations should carry these standards out 'In the spirit of, as well as to the letter of, the law in the public interest, to high ethical standards, achieving value for money.'

Together, the Nolan principles and Treasury standards provide a blueprint for the underlying culture and values of every public sector organisation.

The NHS Constitution

Since January 2010 all providers and commissioners of NHS-funded care have had a statutory duty to have regard to the *NHS Constitution* in all their decisions and actions. As the Department of Health's website states: 'This means that the Constitution, its pledges, principles, values and responsibilities need to be fully embedded and ingrained into everything the NHS does.'

Of particular note in governance terms are the principles and values set out in the Constitution as these need to underpin everything that an organisation does.

NHS Constitution

Principles

- The NHS provides a comprehensive service, available to all
- Access to NHS services is based on clinical need, not an individual's ability to pay
- The NHS aspires to the highest standards of excellence and professionalism
- NHS services must reflect the needs and preferences of patients, their families and carers
- The NHS works across organisational boundaries and in partnership with other organisations in the interests of patients, local communities and the wider population
- The NHS is committed to providing best value for taxpayers' money and the most effective, fair and sustainable use of finite resources
- The NHS is accountable to the public, communities and patients that it serves

Values

- Respect and dignity
- Commitment to quality of care
- Compassion
- Improving lives
- Working together for patients
- Everyone counts

Codes of practice

Since the early 1990s, a number of Codes of Practice[3] have been issued to provide practical guidance on governance arrangements. For the most part, the content of these Codes has now been incorporated into legislation. However, for those organisations (for example, non-foundation NHS trusts) which were established prior to the changes in legislation, the Codes may still be relevant. For example, the NHS TDA expects Chairpersons and non-executive directors of non-foundation trusts to subscribe to the *Code of Conduct: Code of Accountability for NHS Boards*, first issued in 1994 and most recently revised in 2013.

---

[3] For example, the *Code of Business Conduct (Standards of Business Conduct for NHS Staff)* (1993); the *Code of Practice on Openness in the NHS* (2003) and the *Code of Conduct for NHS Managers* (2002).

Bribery Act

The *Bribery Act 2010* applies to both organisations and individuals and means that NHS bodies must ensure that they have in place adequate procedures to prevent bribery taking place. If they fail to do this, organisations can be prosecuted for the failure to prevent a bribe being paid on the organisation's behalf (for example when placing a contract for a major service or investment).

Freedom of Information Act

The *Freedom of Information Act 2000* means that NHS bodies are required to answer questions from members of the public and make information available to them. In addition, the Government has introduced new requirements in relation to transparency which requires the publication of items of spend over £25,000.

Structures and Processes

Organisational structures

The Government (via the Secretary of State, the Department of Health and NHS England) sets down key structures that NHS organisations must have in place. The only exception is foundation trusts (FTs) where structures are set by Monitor.

Although these structures vary according to the type of organisation, two basic principles apply to all – each must have its own governing body (often called the Board) and a designated 'Accountable' (or 'Accounting') Officer. In addition:

- FTs have a Council of Governors that is representative of the local community. Governors can be elected or appointed and do not get involved with the FT's day-to-day running – instead their key role is to hold the FT's Board of Directors to account for the FT's performance and (when necessary) challenge the directors
- CCGs have a Council of Members that is made up of a member (or members) from each constituent GP practice. This Council then delegates functions to the governing body (and to its members; employees; committees or sub-committees).

The governing body – purpose

An NHS organisation's governing body is responsible for the strategies and actions of the organisation (including meeting its statutory duties) and is accountable to the public, Secretary of State and Parliament. Its prime duty is to 'add value to the organisation, enabling it to deliver healthcare and health improvement within the law and without causing harm. It does this by providing a framework within which the organisation can thrive and grow'.[4] In practice, this means that the governing body sets the strategy and objectives for the organisation, monitors their achievement, and looks for potential problems and risks that might prevent them achieving those objectives. The governing body also receives assurances about whether things are working as they should.

---

[4] *Governing the NHS: a Guide for NHS Boards*, Department of Health and the (then) Appointments Commission, 2003.

Given its status and role, there is a range of responsibilities and decisions that the governing body cannot delegate. These are referred to as being 'reserved to the Board'.

> **Examples of Activities 'Reserved to the Board'**
> - Financial stewardship responsibilities (for example, adopting the annual report and accounts that all NHS bodies are required to produce)
> - Determining the organisation's strategy and policies and setting its strategic direction
> - Appointing senior executives
> - Overseeing the delivery of services
> - Standards of governance and behaviour

In addition, an NHS organisation's governing body is free to agree other issues that only it will deal with and must also decide which responsibilities it will delegate by drawing up a scheme of delegation.

As noted above, the situation for CCGs is different as the Council of Members 'sits above' the CCG's governing body and delegates functions to it. At the same time the legislation (and section 6.6 of NHS England's guidance on CCG model constitutions) requires the CCG governing body (not the Council of Members) to appoint the audit and remuneration committees, and to be responsible for (inter alia):

- 'ensuring that the group has appropriate arrangements in place to exercise its functions effectively, efficiently and economically and in accordance with the group's principles of good governance (its main function)
- determining the remuneration, fees and other allowances payable to employees or other persons providing services to the group and the allowances payable under any pension scheme
- approving any functions of the group that are specified in regulations
- other functions delegated to it by the CCG.'

This means that for CCGs, the pre-eminent body is formally the Council of Members. However, in practice the Council delegates functions to its governing body which then operates in much the same way and with the same objectives as other NHS organisations' governing bodies.

The governing body – composition

All NHS bodies are required to have a governing body (or Board) which comprises both executive and non-executive directors (NEDs). This Board is separate from the day-to-day management structure. The exact structure of each Board is different for each type of NHS body and is set out in legislation and associated regulations.[5]

---

[5] For non-foundation NHS trusts: regulations 2 and 4 of the *1990 Trust Membership and Procedure Regulations (SI 1990/2024)*. For FTs: schedule 7 to the *NHS Act 2006*. For CCGs: s14L of the *NHS Act 2006* (inserted by s25 of the 2012 Act) and the associated regulations (SI 2012/1631).

The **Boards of both non-foundation trusts and FTs** comprise a Chair, executive members (who are employees of the NHS organisation) and independent NEDs. The executive directors must include a medical director and nursing director as well as the Chief Executive and Chief Finance Officer (CFO).

CCG governing bodies must include at least two independent lay members (equivalent to NEDs), at least one registered nurse and a doctor who is a secondary care specialist. The CCG's Chief Executive and CFO must also be members of the governing body. The two lay members have specific responsibilities: one has a lead role in patient and public involvement, while the other oversees key elements of the governance arrangements including audit. In addition, one of the lay members undertakes the role of the governing body's Chairperson or the Deputy Chairperson.

NEDs and lay members play a particularly important role on the governing body as they provide independent, constructive challenge and a breadth of experience. By balancing the views of executive directors, they also ensure that power is not concentrated in a few hands so preventing any individual or small group from dominating the governing body's decision making.

The governing body – appointments

Since April 2013, responsibility for appointing, re-appointing (and where necessary terminating) Chairs and NEDs to the governing bodies of non-foundation NHS trusts has rested with the NHS Trust Development Authority (NHS TDA). CCG lay appointments must be approved by NHS England. FTs are responsible for appointing their own directors and Monitor's *Code of Governance* recommends that a nominations committee is set up (or two separate nominations committees) for executive and non-executive appointments to ensure that independence is enshrined in the process and appointments are made on the basis of the governing body's needs and the individual's ability. Monitor also recommends that the Board of Directors appoint a 'senior independent director' from amongst the NEDs (in consultation with the Council of Governors) so that there is someone to deal with concerns of governors and/or members that cannot be resolved through 'normal channels' (i.e. via the Chairperson, the Chief Executive, or CFO).

Governing body committees

To help a governing body discharge its duties effectively, a number of committees are normally established so that it can focus on strategic issues, whilst maintaining arrangements for robust review, scrutiny and challenge of information. It is up to each organisation to decide what committee structure best suits its needs. However, there are two mandatory committees – audit and remuneration.

Audit committee

Every NHS organisation must have an audit committee that reports to the governing body. This committee's distinctive characteristic is that it comprises only independent non-executive members – there is usually at least three, to allow for a quorum of two. In addition, the

Chairperson of the organisation should not be a member. The fact that only non-executives can be members allows the audit committee to operate independently of executive management and to be objective when scrutinising the arrangements put in place and operated by the organisation's executive.

For CCGs, schedule 2, paragraph 7(3) of the *Health and Social Care Act 2012* says that 'Arrangements...**may** include provision for the audit committee to include individuals who are not members of the governing body.' However, NHS England's model constitution for CCGs recommends that they should follow the *Audit Committee Handbook* which makes clear that audit committees should be (and be seen to be) independent and comprise 'not less than three non-executive directors, with a quorum of two'.

The Chief Executive and all other executive directors attend whenever they are invited by the audit committee Chairperson and, in particular, to provide assurances and explanations to the committee when it is discussing audit reports or other matters within their areas of responsibility.

Detailed guidance about the role of audit committees is set out in the *Audit Committee Handbook* which is available from the HFMA and Department of Health websites. However, the Handbook makes clear that one of the committee's key duties is to 'review the establishment and maintenance of an effective system of integrated governance, risk management and internal control, across the whole of the organisation's activities (both clinical and non-clinical), that supports the achievement of the organisation's objectives'.

Remuneration committee

The remuneration (and terms of service) committee reports to the governing body and advises it about the pay, other benefits and terms of employment for the Chief Executive and other senior staff. To ensure that people involved in the day-to-day running of the organisation do not make sensitive decisions, the committee's membership comprises the organisation's Chairperson and at least two other NEDs. The Chief Executive and Human Resources Director may attend other than when his or her own position is being considered. In CCGs, membership must be drawn from the governing body with one acting as the committee's Chairperson. Individuals who claim a significant proportion of their income from the CCG should not be members and member practices should not be in the majority.

Accountable/Accounting Officers

Every NHS organisation has an 'Accountable' (or 'Accounting') Officer.[6] This is a formal role conferred upon the organisation's 'Chief Officer' (usually the Chief Executive). In a CCG, the Chief Officer is either the 'lead manager' or the 'lead clinician.'

Being the Accountable (or Accounting) Officer, means that the nominated individual is accountable to:

---

[6] It is possible for organisations to share senior posts (including an Accountable Officer) providing there are clear agreements about roles and responsibilities and that potential conflicts of interest are declared and managed.

- the organisation's governing body for meeting the objectives it sets, for day-to-day management and for ensuring that governance arrangements are effective
- Parliament/the Department of Health/NHS TDA/NHS England for the proper stewardship of public money and assets and for the organisation's performance.

The duties of Accountable/Accounting Officers are set out in detail in memoranda issued by either: the Department of Health; Monitor (for FTs); the NHS TDA (for non-foundation NHS trusts); NHS England (for CCGs). The memorandum is signed by the nominated individual.

Accountable/Accounting Officers' key duties are to make sure that their organisations:

- operate effectively, economically and with probity
- use their resources prudently and economically, avoiding waste and extravagance
- keep proper accounts.

The role of the Accountable/Accounting Officer is a key element in governance terms with a line of accountability stretching up to Parliament. For non-foundation NHS trusts, Accountable Officers are accountable to the NHS TDA's Accountable Officer who is in turn accountable to the Department of Health's Accounting Officer (and on to the Secretary of State and Parliament). For FTs, Accounting Officers are accountable directly to Parliament (with Monitor providing regulatory oversight).[7]

The position for CCGs is different as they select their own Accountable Officers. However, the individual must then be appointed formally by NHS England at the time of authorisation. Also, if CCGs choose to share an Accountable Officer with another CCG, there must be a joint memorandum of understanding and approval by NHS England during the authorisation process.

Lines of Accountability

CCGs

Parliament
↑
Secretary of State for Health (via Department of Health Accounting Officer)
↑
NHS England Accounting Officer
↑
CCG Accountable officer

---

[7] This is the reason for the two slightly different terms – an Accounting Officer (for example in an FT or Department of Health) is directly accountable to Parliament (via the Public Accounts Committee) but an Accountable Officer (for example, in a CCG or NHS trust) is responsible to an Accounting Officer of a government department who is in turn accountable to Parliament.

Non-foundation NHS Trusts

Parliament
↑
Secretary of State for Health
↑
Department of Health Accounting Officer
↑
NHS Trust Development Authority Accountable Officer
↑
NHS Trust Accountable Officer

Foundation Trusts

Parliament
↑
NHS Foundation Trust Accounting Officer

CCG Accountable Officers' responsibilities are set out in NHS England's guidance *Clinical Commissioning Group Governing Body Members: Role Outlines, Attributes and Skills*. This *states* that the Accountable Officer is charged with ensuring that their CCG 'complies with its:

- duty to exercise its functions effectively, efficiently and economically
- duty to exercise its functions with a view to securing continuous improvement in the quality of services provided to individuals for, or in connection with, the prevention, diagnosis or treatment of illness
- financial obligations, including information requests
- obligations relating to accounting and auditing
- duty to provide information to NHS England, following requests from the Secretary of State.'

Chief Finance Officers

CFOs (also called Finance Directors or Directors of Finance) of health organisations are automatically executive directors with a seat on the governing body. This is in line with the Treasury's guide, *Managing Public Money* which states that the CFO should 'have Board status equivalent to other Board members' and that he or she should be 'a member of the senior leadership team'. Where a CFO fulfils the role for more than one organisation, he or she must be on the governing body of each organisation.

The HFMA has issued a policy statement on the *Role of the CFO in the NHS* which looks at the role in more detail.

Executive management

Each NHS organisation must have an effective management structure designed to achieve its statutory duties and implement the strategic objectives and policies agreed by the governing body. This structure will vary between organisations but should ensure that all areas of responsibility are clearly accountable to a manager and ultimately to an executive director.

Organisational processes

As well as ensuring that an organisation's structure is in line with statutory requirements and that governing bodies are able to monitor, respond and adhere to legislative and regulatory developments, the delivery of healthcare depends on effective internal procedures and controls. Collectively these are sometimes referred to as 'business rules' – key elements that NHS organisations need to think about in relation to finance are:

- effective Board reporting
- standing orders
- procedures for dealing with any conflicts of interest
- standing financial instructions/prime financial policies
- policies and procedures.

Governing body reports

Governing bodies must ensure that they receive sufficient regular financial (and non-financial) information in a succinct and efficient form to enable them to fulfil their responsibilities, monitor progress towards achieving agreed strategies and make informed decisions. Although it is for the Board to decide the form and content of these reports they must ensure that all key areas of activity are covered and that links to strategic objectives are clear. The purpose of a report should also be clear – this can be achieved by including a covering sheet that describes:

- why the report is being presented to the governing body
- how it links with either statutory duties or strategic objectives
- what the governing body is expected to do with it (i.e. is it for decision, approval, or information?).

The Doctor Foster publication *The Intelligent Board* suggests that 'the key tests of the success of any information resource for the Board will be the extent to which it:

- prompts relevant and constructive challenge
- supports informed decision-making
- is effective in providing early warning of potential financial or other problems
- develops all directors' understanding of the organisation and its performance.'

Standing orders

All NHS organisations must have standing orders (SOs) which provide a comprehensive framework for carrying out activities and are therefore a critical element in the governance framework. Effectively, SOs are the link to an organisation's statutory powers and translate these powers into a series of practical rules designed to protect the interests of both the organisation and its staff. In many ways SOs are similar to the memorandum and articles of association of a company. In FTs and CCGs, SOs form part of the constitution.

What Standing Orders Contain

The majority of provisions within SOs relate to the business of running the governing body and structure of its committees – for example:

* the composition of the Board and committees
* how meetings are run
* form, content and frequency of reports
* what constitutes a quorum
* record of attendance
* voting procedures.

Other areas covered include:

* appointment of committees and sub–committees
* scheme of delegation – a detailed listing of what the governing body alone can decide on and who it empowers to take actions or make decisions on its behalf
* decisions reserved to the Board – those decisions that the governing body cannot delegate
* standards of business conduct – for example, relating to how contracts should be awarded to prevent bias or the circumstances under which commercial sponsorship is acceptable
* declarations of interest
* register of interests and hospitality
* duties and obligations of Board members.

Conflicts of interest

One area covered by SOs that often receives particular attention relates to **standards of business conduct, declarations of interest and registers of interests/hospitality**. Chairs and governing body/Board directors must declare any personal or business interests or relationships that may influence (or be perceived to influence) their judgement or decisions. The fundamental principle is that no one should use their public position for private gain, either for their own benefit or for the benefit of those close to them. For example, if a governing body member or member of staff has any interest in a contract, that interest must be disclosed and they must take no part in the evaluation process or decision.

It is important that both actual and potential conflicts of interest are declared as any outside interest, hospitality or sponsorship represents a risk of a conflict arising. The procedures followed to manage conflicts of interest also help protect individuals from any subsequent allegations of bias. The *Bribery Act 2010* also makes it an offence to accept gifts or hospitality as an inducement or reward for doing something in your public role and staff are advised to refuse to accept such gifts or hospitality rather than declare them subsequently. There is usually some leeway for minor gifts (for example, pens or diaries) but the offer of higher value items should be questioned. The key point here is that governing body members and staff must be open about any gifts they have received or been offered. A good test is to think about how it would look on the front page of the local newspaper: if the action or gift could not be defended then it should not be carried out or accepted.

Standing financial instructions (SFIs)/prime financial policies (PFPs)

SFIs/PFPs cover financial aspects in more depth and set out detailed procedures and responsibilities. They are designed to ensure that NHS organisations account fully and openly for all that they do. Although FTs are not required to have SFIs/PFPs, many do and others have written financial procedures that fulfil the same function.

Other policies and procedures

For NHS bodies to run smoothly and effectively, many more policies and procedures (both financial and non-financial) are required, all of which contribute to the achievement of the organisation's overarching objectives. These policies and procedures are usually pulled together in manuals and made available to all staff via the organisation's intranet. These cover a wide variety of areas including:

* financial – for example, banking procedures, use of credit cards
* corporate – for example, health and safety, information systems, research protocols and equal opportunities
* clinical – systems to ensure that the quality of clinical services is continually improved and high standards of care safeguarded. For example, protocols for nursing care, prescribed routines in pharmacy departments and checklists for surgery (collectively these systems are referred to as 'clinical governance').

Control Frameworks

As well as sound structures and processes, organisations also need an effective and comprehensive system of internal control that can provide an assurance to the governing body (and other stakeholders) that things are running as they should. An effective internal control system is based on a structured approach to identifying key strategic organisational objectives, risks that could prevent them from being achieved and the potential impact if those risks are realised. The key mechanisms used to ensure that this happens in practice are collectively referred to as the organisation's 'assurance framework'.

Assurance framework

The assurance framework is usually summarised and brought together for review by the governing body in a single document which is described in the *NHS Audit Committee Handbook* as 'the key source of evidence that links strategic objectives to risks, controls and assurances, and the main tool that the Board should use in discharging its overall responsibility for internal control'.

Each organisation designs its own 'assurance framework' (sometimes referred to as a 'Board Assurance Framework' or BAF) based on a sound understanding of the principal risks (clinical, financial and business) that could prevent it from achieving its agreed objectives and the potential effect each risk could present to those objectives. To help governing bodies do this, the Department of Health issued *Building an Assurance framework: a Practical Guide* which defines a number of essential steps.

How to Build an Assurance Framework

1. Establish strategic objectives
2. Identify the principal (or strategic) risks that may threaten the achievement of these objectives
3. Identify and evaluate the design of key controls intended to manage these principal risks
4. Identify the arrangements for obtaining assurance on the effectiveness of these key controls
5. Evaluate the reliability of the assurances identified
6. Identify positive assurances and areas where there are gaps in controls and/or assurances
7. Put in place plans to take corrective action where gaps in controls and/or assurances have been identified in relation to principal risks
8. Maintain dynamic risk management arrangements including, crucially, a well-founded risk register

Risk management

Risk management is all to do with being aware of potential problems, thinking through what effect they could have and planning ahead to prevent them arising. In this context it is important to recognise that no approach to managing risks can give an absolute guarantee that nothing will ever go wrong. Risk is also about opportunities as well as threats. Good risk management encourages organisations to take well-managed risks that allow safe improvement, development, growth and change.

Internal audit

All NHS bodies are required to have an internal audit function that plays a key role in assurance by providing an independent and objective opinion to the Accountable/ Accounting Officer, governing body and audit committee on the extent to which risk management, control and governance arrangements support the aims of the organisation. Each year the Head of Internal Audit must produce an opinion that is used by the Accountable/Accounting Officer to inform the annual governance statement. This statement forms part of each organisation's annual accounts and draws together 'position statements and evidence on governance, risk management and control, to provide a more coherent and consistent reporting mechanism'. See chapter 11 for more details about this statement and the annual accounts.

Healthcare quality outcomes and registration standards

A key consideration in the overall risk management and assurance framework for the NHS is the need to deliver required quality outcomes and achieve pre-set standards of service and safety designed to underpin the delivery of high quality healthcare. The *Health and Social Care*

(*Community Health and Standards*) *Act 2003* established the power for the Secretary of State for Health to set standards. Other key requirements are set by:

- the Care Quality Commission (CQC) – since April 2010, NHS providers have been required to register with the CQC. This process is designed to ensure that people receive services that meet the CQC's essential standards of quality and safety which are also designed to ensure that patients' dignity is respected and their rights protected. The system is focused on outcomes rather than systems and processes and places the views and experiences of people who use services at its centre (see chapter 12)
- the National Institute for Health and Care Excellence (NICE) which issues guidance relating to standards to be followed for specific conditions/treatments
- the Department of Health/NHS England and NHS TDA – health and service priorities for the year ahead are set out in their annual operational plans (see chapter 14).

Clinical audit

Another important element of the overall risk management and assurance framework is clinical audit – a process that is carried out by healthcare professionals themselves and involves:

- setting standards
- measuring current practice
- comparing results with standards
- changing the way things are done
- re-auditing to make sure practice has improved.

In its guide – *Best Practice in Clinical Audit* – NICE states that it sees clinical audit as being 'the component of clinical governance that offers the greatest potential to assess the quality of care routinely provided for NHS users' and that it (clinical audit) 'should therefore be at the very heart of clinical governance systems'.

For NHS governing bodies, managing clinical risk is just as important (if not more so) as managing financial and business risk. Good clinical audit is, therefore, an enormous asset and source of assurance. In addition, organisations are required to declare their participation in clinical audit in the annual quality accounts (see chapter 11).

For more about clinical audit see *Clinical Audit: a simple guide for NHS Boards*, published by the Healthcare Quality Improvement Partnership in 2010.

Counter fraud and corruption

The emphasis on dealing with fraud and corruption in the NHS has increased significantly over recent years. This is reflected in the fact that section 6 of the general conditions of the *NHS Standard Contract 2013/14* requires provider organisations to put in place and maintain adequate counter fraud and security arrangements. Within one month of service commencement, the provider must complete a crime risk assessment using the applicable toolkit provided by NHS Protect and in accordance with NHS guidance. Following its completion, the provider must take the necessary action to meet the standards set by NHS

Protect at the level indicated by the completed crime risk profile. The standards cover the areas of:

- strategic governance
- inform and involve
- prevent and deter
- hold to account.

CCGs are also required to have access to 'appropriate, accredited counter fraud support' and the publication *Clinical Commissioning Group Guide for Applicants*, clearly states in criterion 4.2 that CCGs must be able to deliver all their statutory functions including strategic oversight, quality improvement, financial control and probity. Therefore CCGs are expected to co-operate with NHS Protect and its nominated officers in the discharge of its functions, such as allowing NHS Protect access to CCG premises, members, employees, documents and information in relation to the promotion of counter fraud measures.

Both counter fraud and security management in the NHS are overseen by NHS Protect which is part of the NHS Business Services Agency. Its role is to lead on identifying and tackling crime across the NHS – for more details, see its website. In addition, NHS Protect hosts a National Fraud Reporting Hotline.

NHS Litigation Authority (NHS LA)

The NHS LA is an arm's length body of the Department of Health and plays an important role in relation to risk management. It was established as a special health authority in 1995 to manage negligence and other claims against the NHS in England on behalf of its member organisations. Since April 2013 this has included independent sector providers of NHS care. The NHS LA runs the clinical negligence scheme for trusts (CNST) which involves the NHS LA assessing its members on the basis of a set of risk management standards that are designed to focus on aspects that are known to affect outcomes and the rate of claims.

Key Learning Points

- The three fundamental principles of governance are openness, integrity and accountability
- An effective approach to governance should underpin everything that an organisation does
- Clinical scandals have shown clear links to governance failings – if an NHS organisation gets its approach to governance wrong it can have a catastrophic impact
- There are three key elements to governance – culture and values; policies, structures and processes; control frameworks
- Good leadership and management are crucial to sound governance as is a shared ethos or culture and a 'tone' that is set from the top
- Everyone who works in the public sector should adhere to the seven principles of public life
- The principles and values set out in the NHS Constitution should underpin all that an organisation does

- Every NHS organisation must have a governing body, audit and remuneration committees, an Accountable/Accounting Officer and a Chief Finance Officer
- The governing body (which includes both executive and non-executive members) is responsible for the strategies and actions of the organisation and is ultimately accountable to the public and Parliament
- One of the audit committee's key roles is to review the system of integrated governance, risk management and internal control across the whole of the organisation's activities
- The remuneration committee advises the governing body about pay, benefits and terms of employment of senior staff
- The Accountable/Accounting Officer is accountable to the organisation and (ultimately) to Parliament
- CFOs are automatically executive directors with a seat on the governing body
- Standing orders provide a framework for carrying out activities and translate statutory powers and duties into practical rules that all must abide by
- Organisations need an effective and comprehensive system of internal control that provides an assurance that things are running as they should
- All NHS organisations must have clear objectives and an understanding of the risks that could prevent their achievement, the possible impact and how they can be avoided
- An assurance framework links key objectives and risks with the main sources of assurance used by the Board to ensure effective internal control
- Managing clinical risk is just as important (if not more so) as financial and business risk – clinical audit is therefore a key source of assurance in this area
- Counter fraud and security management are overseen by NHS Protect.

References and Further Reading

Introductory Guide to Governance in the NHS, HFMA, 2011:
www.hfma.org.uk/publications-and-guidance/publicationitem.htm?publicationid=56&catid=2

The Financial Aspects of Corporate Governance (the Cadbury Committee Report, 1992):
www.ecgi.org/codes/code.php?code_id=132

The Mid Staffordshire NHS Foundation Trust Inquiry (the Francis Report):
www.midstaffsinquiry.com/pressrelease.html

Quality Governance in the NHS - A guide for provider boards, National Quality Board (Department of Health), 2011: https://www.gov.uk/government/publications/quality-governance-in-the-nhs-a-guide-for-provider-boards

Taking it on Trust – a review of how NHS trusts and foundation trusts get their assurance, Audit Commission, 2009:
http://archive.audit-commission.gov.uk/auditcommission/sitecollectiondocuments/AuditCommissionReports/NationalStudies/29042009takingontrustREP.pdf

Leadership Framework, NHS Leadership Academy, 2011:
www.leadershipacademy.nhs.uk/wp-content/uploads/2012/11/NHSLeadership-Leadership-Framework-LF-Quick-Reference-Guide-Summary-of-Domains-Elements-and-Stages.pdf

Good Governance Standard for Public Services, The Independent Commission on Good Governance in Public Services, 2005:
www.jrf.org.uk/publications/good-governance-standard-public-services

Standards for Members of NHS Boards and Clinical Commissioning Group Governing Bodies in England, Professional Standards Authority for Health and Social Care, 2012:
www.professionalstandards.org.uk/docs/psa-library/november-2012—standards-for-board-members.pdf?sfvrsn=0

The Committee on Standards in Public Life (including the 7 'Nolan Principles'):
www.public-standards.gov.uk/

Managing Public Money, HM Treasury: www.hm-treasury.gov.uk/psr_mpm_index.htm

The NHS Constitution: www.gov.uk/government/publications/the-nhs-constitution-for-england

The Code of Conduct: Code of Accountability in the NHS, Department of Health, 2004 and issued in updated form by the NHS TDA in 2013:
www.ntda.nhs.uk/2013/04/26/useful-info-for-non-execs/

Code of Practice on Openness in the NHS, 2003: http://www.cfoi.org.uk/nhscoptext.html

Code of Conduct for NHS Managers, Department of Health (first published in 2002):
www.nhsemployers.org/EmploymentPolicyAndPractice/UKEmploymentPractice/Pages/Core-Standards-For-NHS-Managers.aspx

Standards of Business Conduct for NHS Staff, Department of Health, 1993 (archived web pages):
http://webarchive.nationalarchives.gov.uk/+/www.dh.gov.uk/en/Publicationsandstatistics/Lettersandcirculars/Healthserviceguidelines/DH_4017845

Model Constitution Framework for CCGs, NHS England, 2012:
www.commissioningboard.nhs.uk/resources/resources-for-ccgs/ccg-mod-cons-framework/

Monitor (including the Governance and Audit Codes for NHS Foundation Trusts, reference guide for governors and the Accounting Officer memorandum): www.monitor-nhsft.gov.uk

Health and Social Care Act 2012: www.legislation.gov.uk/ukpga/2012/7/contents/enacted

NHS Audit Committee Handbook, HFMA, 2011:
www.hfma.org.uk/publications-and-guidance/publicationitem.htm?publicationid=52&catid=2

Accountable Officer Memorandum, Department of Health:
www.info.doh.gov.uk/doh/finman.nsf/072561aa006322660725618c006b09a0/886b090cc16e3435802568f70038d71d?OpenDocument

Clinical Commissioning Group Governing Body Members: Role Outlines, Attributes and Skills, NHS England, 2012: www.commissioningboard.nhs.uk/files/2012/04/ccg-mem-roles.pdf

The Role of the Chief Finance Officer in the NHS, HFMA: www.hfma.org.uk

The Intelligent Board, Doctor Foster, 2006: http://drfosterintelligence.co.uk/thought-leadership/intelligent-board/

Building an Assurance Framework: A Practical Guide, Department of Health 2003 (archived web pages): http://webarchive.nationalarchives.gov.uk/+/www.dh.gov.uk/en/Publicationsandstatistics/Publications/PublicationsPolicyAndGuidance/DH_4093992

National Institute for Health and Care Excellence (NICE): www.nice.org.uk/

Care Quality Commission: www.cqc.org.uk/

Principles for Best Practice in Clinical Audit – NICE, 2008: www.nice.org.uk/usingguidance/implementationtools/auditadvice/audit_advice.jsp?domedia=1&mid=79613703-19B9-E0B5-D4F14A0429022FC0

Clinical Audit: a Simple Guide for NHS Boards, HQIP, 2010: http://good-governance.org.uk/Products/clinical-audit—simple-guide-for-nhs-boards.htm

NHS Protect: www.nhsprotect.nhs.uk

NHS Protect National Fraud Hotline: 0800 028 40 60

NHS Litigation Authority: www.nhsla.com/Pages/Home.aspx

Chapter 14: Revenue Planning and Budgeting

Overview

NHS organisations are responsible for spending taxpayers' money to ensure that patients have access to high quality care, free at the point of need. As this is taxpayers' money there is an absolute requirement to demonstrate that the money is used well and for its intended purpose. Every NHS organisation also has a specific statutory duty to make 'proper arrangements for securing economy, efficiency and effectiveness in its use of resources'.[1] To be able to meet this requirement, each organisation needs to plan the activities it will deliver or commission and establish the associated resource implications – not just in terms of money but also in relation to staffing, equipment, supplies and so on.

Planning and budgeting takes place in two areas – revenue and capital – which are then brought together in an overall plan. This chapter focuses on the revenue side – in other words, how NHS organisations plan and budget for their day-to-day activities. Capital planning is covered in chapter 15.

Why is Revenue Planning and Budgeting Important?

Revenue planning and budgeting is an integral part of an organisation's business planning process and helps it by establishing:

- an agreed way ahead
- key aims and objectives
- how those aims will be achieved and by when
- a framework for day-to-day operations and decisions.

What the Planning Process involves – Key Documents

The planning process is designed to facilitate the efficient and effective delivery of high quality services, demonstrate accountability and ensure consistency with national and local commissioning plans, targets and outcomes frameworks. There are four key documents:

- a long term (usually 3 to 5 years) strategic **business plan** for the organisation (sometimes referred to as the integrated business plan or IBP)
- a **long term financial plan** that looks at best and 'downside' case scenarios
- an **annual operational/activity plan** that outlines expected activities for the year ahead and shows how the organisation intends to meet its strategic aims
- an **annual financial plan** that sets out the overall budget for the year.

---

[1] Section 26 of the *NHS Act 2006*.

Business plan

The business plan is the written end product of a process that identifies the aims, objectives and resource requirements of an organisation over a three to five year period. It is a detailed document that sets out the assumptions that underlie service plans and budgets for the period covered.

> **What a Business Plan includes**
>
> - An activity and income plan
> - Details of planned service developments
> - Savings or cost improvement plans
> - Performance measures
> - Workforce implications
> - A strategy for the organisation's support services (for example, the estate and information technology)
> - An analysis of the needs and priorities of the wider health community and how and where the organisation fits in

The business plan is considered and approved by the organisation's governing body and then used as a benchmark against which to measure progress towards achieving the organisation's aims and objectives. In practice, this means that the business plan is kept under constant review and updated to reflect the impact of external changes (for example, Government announcements) and internal developments (for example, new clinical techniques).

Long term financial plan

Accompanying the business plan, a long term financial plan is used by NHS organisations to look at the financial impact of achieving their goals over the medium to long term (again over a three to five year period). This plan focuses on the assumptions made in the business plan and enables the organisation to see how potential changes (for example, in local demographics) could affect financial viability. The long term financial plan also includes an analysis of best and 'downside' case scenarios – enabling the organisation to anticipate what might happen if things don't go as planned and have in place strategies to mitigate the impact.

Operational/activity plan

Operational (or activity) plans show how national targets (for example as set out in the *NHS Constitution*) and local priorities (for example, as set out in Joint Health and Wellbeing Strategies and Joint Strategic Needs Assessments developed by Health and Wellbeing Boards – see chapter 8) will be delivered within available resources. They are used by commissioners to outline how they intend to address health inequalities, improve health outcomes and better focus healthcare provision in line with commissioning intentions and strategies. For providers, the focus of an operational plan is how they will deliver the contracts agreed with commissioners and meet their own objectives and priorities (for example, the need to achieve required cost improvements or carry out service re-design).

Operational plans are reviewed regularly throughout the year and if significant issues arise that affect progress, adjustments are made – for example, if serious financial problems develop in the health economy.

Annual financial plan/budget

Alongside the operational/activity plan, all NHS organisations must produce an annual financial plan (usually referred to as the budget) that shows the expected revenue and costs of its planned activities for the coming year (both revenue and capital) and demonstrates that the organisation will achieve its financial duties. Chapter 11 looks in detail at these duties but in relation to the budget, the key statutory requirement for non-foundation trusts and commissioners is that they must not spend more money than they have coming in – in other words, they must break even (achieve a 'balanced budget') or deliver a surplus. NHS foundation trusts do not have a statutory duty to break-even but need to remain solvent if they are to continue as going concerns.

To assess the financial position accurately, the budget must cover all expected sources of income and expenditure across the full range of activities for which the organisation is responsible and take account of other non-financial information such as activity levels, savings schemes and staffing requirements. The budget is approved by the governing body and is then used to monitor progress and performance throughout the year so that an organisation knows how much income it is receiving, what it is spending and how much it is overspending or saving at any point in time.

For commissioners, the expenditure side of the budget is based on the activity levels that they have commissioned from providers to meet their commissioning intentions. For providers, the expenditure budget is based on the capacity and workforce they need to have available to meet these levels of activity – this will include the costs of running a service, department or organisation on a day-to-day basis (for example, to meet the costs of staff pay, travel expenses, overheads, drugs and other consumables). Providers will also have a budget for income – for example, split between income for patient care activity, teaching and education, and other areas such as research and development activity.

The capital budget is based on plans for major spending on land, buildings, equipment and other durable items that are expected to be used for more than one year and have a value of £5,000 or more. This expenditure is subject to separate funding and regulations – see chapter 15 for details.

Budgeting in Practice

Approaches

Although organisations refer to their 'budget' (singular), it is actually made up of a series of separate budgets for each activity, service, department or practice. Each part of the organisation develops its own financial, workforce and activity plans to indicate how it will use its share of the money to meet needs and priorities within the overall strategy. There are three basic budgeting approaches – historic, zero-based and activity-based. The NHS tends to use a combination of all three.

Approaches to Budgeting

Historic or incremental budgeting – this uses the previous year's budget, adjusted for known savings (for example, as required in cost improvement programmes); cost rises (for example, pay awards and other inflationary factors) and developments (for example, if a new service is introduced or another discontinued or if National Institute for Health and Care Excellence (NICE) prescribing guidance changes). Allowance is also made for the financial consequences of any new policy developments.

Zero-based budgeting – this involves starting with a blank sheet of paper each year and results in a completely fresh financial plan. It tends to be used for the introduction of new services or when activities are under review.

Activity-based budgeting – this approach looks at what drives costs and is linked to activity levels. It requires those involved in setting the budget to know and understand the costs of delivering particular activities and services – for example, being clear about what costs are fixed and those that are variable (i.e. costs that will increase or decrease as activity increases or decreases – see chapter 17 for more on costing). The aim is to ensure that no matter what the actual level of activity, the correct resources are available to fund it.

Budget management

Another important feature of any budget in the NHS is that it is not the sole responsibility of the finance experts. Instead, it is essential to have a single named individual responsible for developing and managing each budget (the 'budget holder' or 'budget manager'). That person uses their knowledge and experience to help develop the budget and has the authority to take decisions relating to it. This means that responsibility for a budget must be aligned with the ability to control income and expenditure (i.e. the ability to take decisions that will incur a cost or result in a flow of income). To be effective a budget holder must understand what needs to be delivered and which organisational, local and national objectives they contribute to.

In practice, this means that each budget is managed at the lowest practicable level by the person who understands the activity or service covered and who is responsible for committing the expenditure. This is what is known as 'devolved budget management'.

Budget monitoring

Once a budget is agreed, it is used by the budget holders to monitor how things are turning out via regular (usually monthly) monitoring. In other words, actual performance is compared with what was planned so that when necessary, corrective action can be taken. For example, there may be an unexpected increase in the cost of equipment or a new initiative may fail to deliver the level of savings expected.

The Planning Process – Key External Constraints

Given that all NHS organisations are statutory bodies, they do not have a free hand when it comes to developing their plans. Instead they must reflect national policy imperatives, meet targets and financial duties set by Government and reflect local priorities. The main factors that directly affect revenue planning are:

- the *NHS Constitution*
- the *NHS Outcomes Framework*
- annual operational guidelines
- efficiency requirements
- QIPP plans
- allocations – the money received from the Treasury via the Department of Health or NHS England
- payment by results guidance
- National Institute for Health and Care Excellence (NICE) guidelines.

The NHS Constitution and the Outcomes Framework

The *NHS Constitution* and the *Outcomes Framework* are key documents for all NHS organisations as they set out overall objectives and responsibilities that apply across the board. Whilst the Constitution's focus is on overarching rights, values and principles (see chapter 13), it also sets out a series of specific pledges – for example, in relation to referral to treatment times, A & E waits, cancelled operations and ambulance response times. The *Outcomes Framework* has a more direct impact on day-to-day planning as it sets out what NHS organisations are expected to achieve in terms of healthcare outcomes for patients across five broad domains. For each domain a number of areas for improvement are identified but there are no set targets associated with them.

Outcomes Framework – the Five Domains

1. Preventing people from dying prematurely.
2. Enhancing quality of life for people with long term conditions.
3. Helping people to recover from episodes of ill-health or following injury.
4. Ensuring people have a positive experience of care.
5. Treating and caring for people in a safe environment and protecting them from avoidable harm.

Annual operational guidelines

As well as the overarching *Outcomes Framework*, annual operational guidelines are issued. Until 2013/14, the key document was the Department of Health's *Operating Framework* which set out in detail what was expected of all NHS organisations each year and in particular the national priorities against which NHS organisations were expected to improve.

For commissioners, this role has now been assumed by NHS England which issued its first annual planning guidance – *Everyone Counts: Planning for Patients 2013/14* – in December 2012. This sets out what NHS England will do in 2013/14 to help clinical commissioning groups (CCGs) deliver improvements to patients and identifies areas that they should focus on relating to each of the five outcome framework domains (see above). There is also a *CCG Outcomes*

Indicator Set 2013/14 which was developed by NICE and is designed to help CCGs 'drive local improvement and set priorities'.

Although specific targets have not been set (other than in relation to reducing clostridium difficile infections), NHS England expects CCGs to 'set out real ambition in their plans', make progress against the domains and 'develop their own local priorities through their input to the Joint Health and Wellbeing Strategy'. Each CCG must report progress to the relevant NHS England area team and identify three priorities against which progress is more closely monitored – improvements in these three areas (as well as against the national measures) will then be used to assess the 'quality premium' paid in the following year.

> ### The Quality Premium
>
> The 'quality premium' rewards CCGs 'for improvements in the quality of the services that they commission and for associated improvements in health outcomes and reducing inequalities'. The premium paid will be based on achievement against four national measures and three local measures.

Detailed guidance (including a timetable for the development of CCG plans) has been issued by NHS England.

As far as providers are concerned, they must take account of commissioners' plans and the local Joint Health and Wellbeing Strategy in developing their own operational plans.

For non-foundation trusts that are working towards foundation status, planning guidelines and detailed technical guidance have been produced by the NHS Trust Development Authority. *Toward High Quality Sustainable Services* emphasises that non-foundation trust plans must show that the organisation has a 'clear strategy to deliver against each of the key areas of quality, finance and performance'. The technical guidance[2] includes details of the submissions required as part of the planning process.

Foundation trusts must submit three-year plans to Monitor each year that set out their financial and strategic plans. Detailed guidance for the financial commentary that these plans include and a template is issued by Monitor – see its website for details.

Efficiency requirements

The NHS budget is now growing at a much slower rate than over recent years but demand for its services continues to rise. At the same time the Department of Health has set an overall savings target for the NHS of £20 billion over four years (i.e. by 2014/15).[3] In practice, this means that every NHS organisation needs to deliver on average 4% of on-going 'efficiencies'

---

[2] *Toward High Quality, Sustainable Services: Technical Guidance for Operating Plans*, NHS TDA, December 2012.

[3] The so-called 'Nicholson Challenge' as it was David Nicholson, then the Chief Executive of the NHS who set the target.

every year (i.e. they must make savings by doing what they do more cost effectively) and reflect this in their annual financial plans.

At a more detailed level, if the cost of an organisation's plans to purchase and/or deliver services exceeds its anticipated levels of income, savings must be included within the budget to bring it back in line with the available resources.

QIPP plans

To help achieve efficiency targets whilst maintaining and improving quality, the Department of Health introduced the 'quality, innovation, productivity and prevention (QIPP) challenge'. In practice, this means organisations follow the 'lean management principles' of avoiding duplication, preventing errors that need to be corrected, and stopping ineffective practices. International evidence has shown that it is possible to improve the quality of care and patient experience while reducing costs. CCGs are responsible for leading the QIPP agenda (supported by NHS England) but all NHS organisations have a role to play in its delivery. This is made clear in NHS England's guidelines *Everyone Counts: Planning for Patients 2013/14* which states that although provider organisations must ensure that their cost improvement programmes do not have a negative impact on service quality, CCGs must also carry out their own assessments and 'be satisfied that services are safe for patients with no reduction in quality.' To help them do this the guidance tells CCGs they should use a number of resources including the National Quality Board's 'how to guides'.

Allocations

As mentioned earlier in this chapter, all non-foundation NHS organisations must achieve a balanced budget each year (and FTs must remain solvent) and so the income level they receive is of critical importance. For commissioners the key factor is the funding allocation they receive from NHS England and for providers, the income secured through contracts with commissioners. For more about the allocation process and how services are funded, see chapter 10.

Payment by results

Another set of guidelines that both commissioners and providers must take account of when preparing their plans relates to payment by results (PbR). Under PbR, commissioners pay providers a price (or tariff) for each patient seen or treated. The price paid takes account of the relative complexity of the patient's healthcare needs.

The volume of activity covered by PbR amounts to around a third of CCG budgets overall. However, for some acute hospitals, it can drive a significant proportion of income. This activity is difficult to plan for as tariffs can vary significantly between years as a result of three key factors:

- the different levels of efficiency savings included within the tariff (each year the PbR guidance specifies the percentage savings that are built in)
- an adjustment for cost increases

- the use of a more recent set of costs – in the summer of each year, all providers of services to NHS patients funded with NHS money must submit details of activity levels, unit cost data and average lengths of stay for a range of specified activities; this is known as the reference cost submission (see chapter 17 for more details).

A change in tariff between years can also reflect changes in casemix, activity levels, improvements in costing practice and clinical practice. In addition, changes in the PbR 'rules' and the introduction of specific measures to influence the behaviour of NHS organisations can mean that providers are paid significantly more or less than they were for the same activity in the previous year.

As part of the planning process, organisations must also take into account the 'market forces factor' (MFF) which is paid in addition to the national tariff to reflect unavoidable cost differences between organisations (for example, staff costs are higher in London than elsewhere in the country). The MFF is set annually by the Department for each service provider and ranges from 1.00 to nearly 1.30, meaning that the organisation with the highest MFF receives a top-up to the tariff of nearly 30% for all its PbR activity to reflect its higher unavoidable costs.

See chapter 18 for more about PbR and MFF.

NICE guidelines

NICE provides national guidance and advice that is designed to improve the quality of health and social care. Of particular importance in planning terms are its quality standards which its website describes as being 'central to supporting the Government's vision for an NHS and social care system focussed on delivering the best possible outcomes for people who use services'. The standards are developed by NICE in collaboration with relevant professions using a variety of evidence sources.

The standards are reflected in the *Clinical Commissioning Group Outcome Indicator Set* that is designed to help CCGs by providing them with comparative information about the quality of health services commissioned and health outcomes achieved. The *Indicator Set* is published as part of NHS England's annual planning guidance but (as mentioned earlier in this chapter), the announcement makes clear that it does 'not in itself set thresholds or levels of ambition for CCGs, it is intended as a tool for CCGs to drive local improvement and set priorities'.

The quality standards are also used to inform payment mechanisms and incentive schemes such as the Quality and Outcomes Framework (QOF) and Commissioning for Quality and Innovation (CQUIN) – see chapter 6 for more about QOF and chapter 16 for CQUIN.

The Planning Process – Other Influences

As well as reflecting national guidelines in its annual operational plan and budget, an organisation must allow for a range of other factors including, for example:

- service developments (as outlined in its business plan)
- nationally agreed changes to pay and agreed increments for staff
- the impact of changes in clinical practice

- changes in drugs or medical devices used (NICE guidelines are relevant here)
- income streams that are no longer available or received
- changes in national and/or local priorities.

Key Learning Points

- The planning process is designed to ensure efficient and effective delivery of services, demonstrate public accountability and ensure consistency with national and local commissioning plans and targets
- The business plan sets out the assumptions that underlie service plans and budgets
- The operational/activity plan shows how national targets and local priorities will be delivered within the resources available
- Budgets show organisations' expected income and spending levels for the year ahead and demonstrate how their financial duties will be met
- Although organisations refer to **the** budget, it is made up of a series of separate budgets for individual activities or services
- There are three main budgeting approaches (historic, zero-based and activity-based), all of which are used in the NHS
- Budgets are managed by budget holders who monitor actual performance during the year and take corrective action when needed
- When an organisation sets out its plan it must take into consideration both external and internal requirements. Of particular importance are the *NHS Constitution*, the *NHS Outcomes Framework* and annual operational planning guidelines.

References and Further Reading

The NHS Constitution for England, Department of Health, 2013:
www.gov.uk/government/publications/the-nhs-constitution-for-england

The NHS Outcomes Framework 2013/14, Department of Health:
www.gov.uk/government/publications/nhs-outcomes-framework-2013-to-2014

Information and guidance about quality, innovation, productivity and prevention (QIPP), Department of Health:
www.gov.uk/government/policies/making-the-nhs-more-efficient-and-less-bureaucratic

Everyone Counts: Planning for Patients 2013/14, NHS England, 2012:
www.england.nhs.uk/everyonecounts/

CCG Outcomes Indicator Set, NHS England 2013: www.england.nhs.uk/ccg-ois/

NHS England guidance on quality premiums:
www.england.nhs.uk/wp-content/uploads/2013/05/qual-premium.pdf

Toward High Quality, Sustainable Services: Planning Guidance for NHS Trust Boards for 2013/14, NHS TDA, 2012:
www.ntda.nhs.uk/2012/12/21/nhs-tda-publishes-planning-technical-guidance-for-201314/

Monitor guidance on annual plans: www.monitor-nhsft.gov.uk/information-nhs-foundation-trusts/planning-and-reporting-processes/annual-planning

Information about QIPP:
www.improvement.nhs.uk/Default.aspx?alias=www.improvement.nhs.uk/qipp

National Quality Board guidance: http://www.england.nhs.uk/2013/01/24/nqb/

For more about NICE and its guidelines: www.nice.org.uk/

Chapter 15: Capital Funding, Planning and Accounting

> **Overview**
>
> This chapter looks at what capital is and how it is controlled and funded in the NHS. It also runs through the various sources of capital funding and explains how to account for capital assets and changes in their values.

What is Capital in the NHS?

Expenditure is classified as either revenue (spending on day-to-day operations) or capital. Capital spending is incurred when an asset intended for use on a long term basis is acquired – this is also described as capital investment. Specifically, capital assets are defined as:

- being held for delivering services or for administrative purposes
- having a useful life greater than one year
- having a cost which can be measured reliably
- generating future economic benefits or service potential for the organisation.

Capital assets can be both tangible (things that physically exist) and intangible (assets that do not exist as physical entities) – examples are shown below:

Tangible assets	Intangible assets
• Land	• Software licences
• Buildings	• Development costs for software and systems
• Dwellings	
• Assets in the course of construction	• Licences and trademarks
• Plant and machinery	• Patents
• Transport equipment	• Other development costs which may result in an asset
• Information technology (including integral software)	
• Fixtures and fittings	

Asset Registers

Every NHS organisation maintains a register of its assets (tangible and intangible) so that they can be managed effectively and to demonstrate accountability. The register records a range of information about each asset and is used to help in the preparation of the organisation's financial accounts.

> **Asset Registers – what they record for each asset**
>
> * Identification, description and location
> * Date, method of acquisition and initial capital outlay
> * How the asset has been financed (for example, is it owned, leased or covered by a PFI agreement)
> * Opening balance on the 1 April
> * Any additions to the asset
> * The value if reclassified for sale
> * Gains from revaluation (so that there is a clear link to the revaluation reserve – see later in this chapter)
> * Impairments (i.e. a loss in value – see later in this chapter) including any reversals
> * Cumulative depreciation charges and estimated life
> * Closing balance at 31 March

Theoretically, each capital asset should be recorded in the asset register. However, to include all very low value items would be a costly administrative burden. As a result, NHS organisations use a minimum level of expenditure or 'threshold' below which property, plant or equipment is not considered to be a capital asset. Items that fall below this threshold are charged as a revenue cost in the year of purchase and are not recorded in the asset register. The threshold (or 'de minimis level') generally used is £5,000[1] or less (this is the figure set in the Department of Health's *Manual for Accounts*) although this may vary between organisations and should be agreed with the external auditors.

Where assets are interdependent (they only work together) then the de minimis level applies to the cost of the group of assets. An example of grouped assets is IT hardware attached to a network. Groups of similar assets (for example, hospital beds) cannot be grouped together or classed as interdependent as each can be used independently.

The Capital Regime – Allocations, Controls and Limits

Allocations

Overall, the NHS has a capital allocation set by the Treasury (see chapter 10) of approximately £4.4 billion each year. As statutory bodies, all NHS organisations have to work within a statutory and regulatory framework to ensure that this allocation is spent appropriately. This means that there are constraints on the money that they spend.

Clinical commissioning groups (CCGs) are given a capital allocation each year which is based on their 'capital resource limit' (CRL) as set by NHS England. This CRL is used to control their spending (see below for details). However, it is unlikely that CCGs will have significant levels of capital spending as assets that previously belonged to primary care trusts have been transferred to NHS Property Services ltd and it is now responsible for their management (see

---

[1] The £5,000 'threshold' includes VAT where this is not recoverable, installation costs and external fees such as architect, surveyor or installation fees.

chapter 3). Similarly, leases of properties developed under NHS LIFT arrangements have transferred to Community Health Partnerships Ltd (see later in this chapter).

Provider organisations – NHS trusts and foundation trusts (FTs) – are not given a capital allocation so they finance capital expenditure by borrowing or by using internally generated resources. Their controls therefore restrict the amounts that they can use to finance capital expenditure – see below.

Capital resource limit

A CRL is set annually for each relevant organisation and is a statutory duty for commissioners – they should not exceed it and it is monitored throughout the year. Performance against the CRL must be reported in commissioners' annual report and accounts. The organisation should not spend more than its CRL after adjusting for asset disposals and grants and/or donations towards the purchase of capital assets. Underspends against the CRL cannot be carried forward to the following financial year unless they are known in advance and built into submitted plans.

Non-foundation trusts are also given a CRL and are required by the Department of Health (rather than statute) to remain within it. Performance against the CRL is measured in the same way as for commissioners and is also reported in the annual report and accounts. Unlike commissioners, the CRL does not represent the amount of finance given to the trust which is why trusts have other controls to meet.

FTs do not have a CRL.

External financing limit

Non-foundation trusts are also required to remain within their 'external financing limit' (EFL). This was established to control the amount of cash that could be spent on capital in a year. However, since 2008/09, it has been set to include all sources of capital finance, including from:

- the Department of Health (i.e. public dividend capital (PDC)[2] and loans)
- internal generation
- external sources (including finance leases).

This means that the EFL is a 'financing limit' – i.e. the maximum amount of cash that can be accessed through external borrowing. Achievement of the EFL is an **absolute** financial duty. There is no tolerance above the EFL target as it is designed to control the cash expenditure of the NHS as a whole to the level agreed by Parliament. By controlling net cash flows, the EFL sets a limit on the level of cash that an NHS trust may:

- draw from either external sources or its own cash reserves (a positive EFL) **OR**
- repay to external sources for capital borrowing (a negative EFL).

Commissioners and FTs do not have an EFL.

---

[2] PDC is a type of long-term government finance – it is discussed later in the chapter.

Borrowing limits

Prior to the *Health and Social Care Act 2012*,[3] Monitor was required to set a limit on borrowing for each FT. This was set annually using the *Prudential Borrowing Code* which determined how readily capital and working capital could be accessed and the maximum cumulative amount that an FT could borrow. It was set on the assumption that the FT could afford the costs of borrowing to this level both in terms of the interest payments and the repayment of the loan itself, taking into consideration any borrowing it already had.

The 2012 Act establishes new requirements for the Department of Health to produce guidance in relation to the powers that it has to lend to FTs. In this context, lending includes the provision of loans, issue of PDC, giving of grants and any other financial assistance. Monitor's *Risk Assessment Framework* (which applies from mid-2013/14) includes a 'capital servicing capacity ratio' in place of the borrowing limit.

Since 2007/08, non-foundation trusts have been set borrowing limits as well as their EFL and CRL but they can borrow only from the Department of Health – these financing arrangements remain unchanged. The borrowing limit is set in conjunction with the CRL and EFL.

Planning the Capital Programme

There is an absolute requirement when spending public money to demonstrate that it has been used wisely and for its intended purpose. As a result, NHS organisations need to plan, monitor and manage their capital investments.

Affordability

The overriding constraint when planning for capital is that organisations must not spend more than they have available and can afford, both in relation to the capital assets themselves and the associated on-going revenue costs. This means thinking through a number of factors including:

- the need for new infrastructure and strategic developments
- the need to replace medical, IT and other equipment
- maintenance costs
- depreciation costs – capital assets wear out and over their 'useful life' an annual (non-cash) charge is made to the revenue account to reflect this (see later for more about depreciation)
- impact on PDC dividend – this is a cash charge paid to the Department of Health which is based on the average net assets of the organisation. An increase in capital assets results in an increase in the dividend charged (see later in this chapter for more about PDC).

---

[3] Section 163 of the 2012 Act repeals section 41 of the 2006 Act.

Business cases

Under the current regime (2013/14), an NHS organisation has a rolling programme of capital investment to ensure that its asset base is fit for purpose. When additional capital investment is needed, the first stage is usually to develop a business case to consider the options available, their impact and affordability. In the context of capital spending, a business case is a written statement of the need for investment in capital. The business case process is designed to lead to a consideration of changing circumstances, future requirements and opportunities and an agreed corporate view of the best way forward backed up by sound and reasoned assumptions and projections. It is helpful to use a standard format so that key issues are covered.

What a Business Case Includes

The strategic 'fit' of the proposed investment within the local health economy, including a clear and concise statement of need.

Effective project management arrangements, clear lines of communication and details of those key individuals who will be personally accountable.

An indication that the proposal has the support and approval of key stakeholders including commissioners, staff and patients.

Quantified analyses of the investment and its lifetime costs, benefits and cash flows.

Quantified analyses of the costs/benefits of any alternative methods of financing the investment.

Evidence-based information to support the proposal in terms of priority, cost-effectiveness, clinical service management and the best use of scarce resources.

If a major investment is being considered, the business case should also bring together the arguments for the preferred option (including current and future service requirements, affordability, the trust's competitive service position and the ability to complete the project within the specified budget and in line with agreed timescales).

Delegated limits

Business cases for NHS trusts are currently subject to a system of 'delegated limits'. This means that the capital value of a project determines what approvals are required. Non-foundation trusts have a delegated limit for all business cases that is currently £5m or 3% of turnover, whichever is lower (turnover is measured using the trust's previous years financial accounts turnover figure). This means that projects with a capital value of less than £5m (or 3% of turnover) require only the approval of the trust's own governing body or Board. Above this level, external approval is required as shown below.

Delegated Limits for non-foundation NHS trusts	
Financial value of the capital investment	**Approving person or group**
Between £5m or 3% of turnover whichever is lower, and £10m	NHS TDA Director of Finance
£10m to £25m	NHS TDA Capital Investment Group
£25m to £50m	NHS TDA Capital Investment Group AND NHS TDA Board
Over £50m	NHS TDA Capital Investment Group AND NHS TDA Board AND the Department of Health

Source: Delivering High Quality Care for Patients: The Accountability Framework for NHS Trust Boards, NHS TDA, 2013.

CCGs are unable to approve their own business cases.

FTs are not subject to strict limits. However, Monitor's approval is required for significant investments. Whether a project is significant depends on the risks associated with it.

Sources of Capital

The potential sources of funding for capital investments vary by type of NHS organisation.

As mentioned earlier, it is unlikely that CCGs will have significant levels of capital assets as the only source of funding available to them is internally generated funds or any capital allocation given to them by NHS England.

The situation is much clearer for non-foundation trusts and FTs – they have access to a number of well-established funding sources:

- internally generated resources (via retained surpluses, depreciation and proceeds from the sale of capital assets)
- borrowing (including PDC)
- public private partnerships
- leases
- donations and grants.

Internally generated resources

The main source of capital funding is from internally generated resources. In other words, retained surpluses, depreciation and proceeds from the sale of capital assets.

As we mentioned earlier, all NHS bodies must make a charge to the expenditure side of their revenue account to reflect the cost of using an asset over its useful life – this is known as depreciation. This charge does not involve actual cash being paid out (it is 'non-cash') and so an organisation that breaks even or achieves a surplus on its revenue account will generate a cash surplus equivalent to the value of the depreciation charge (all other things being equal). The cash 'generated' and/or any surplus is available to invest in capital projects, such as replacing equipment, enhancing existing assets or building new ones subject to the organisation meeting the capital controls set out earlier in the chapter. It can also be used for revenue purposes – maintenance or sustaining the working capital position.

Another source of finance is the sale of existing assets. While an FT is able to retain the total proceeds from the sale of an asset, the amount of money that a non-foundation trust can retain is capped to match its delegated limit.

Borrowing

The way in which money can be borrowed depends on the type of organisation considering the loan.

To support an investment, non-foundation trusts may borrow from the Department of Health in the form of a capital investment loan (normally interest bearing) which must be linked to specific capital expenditure and local priorities. The loan and its repayments must be affordable and within both the trust's borrowing limit and CRL as noted above. However, it is not generally possible to access the funds until the need arises for the cash – i.e. when the supplier has to be paid for the equipment or the contractor for building works. If the loan is not received in a timely manner, the trust's EFL may be breached – this is a particular risk at year end.

Exceptionally, loans may be approved even if they are not supported by a trust's borrowing limit– for example, where the capital investment itself will lead to future income streams that will enable repayment of the loan.

FTs have greater borrowing freedoms available to them. They have to date been able to borrow from the Foundation Trust Financing Facility (FTFF) as well as from the open market, including commercial loans from banks and other private lending organisations. The FTFF is managed by the Department of Health and interest rates are fixed to the National Loans Fund rate prevailing on the date that the loan agreement is signed.

Investments for non-foundation trusts are channelled through the NHS TDA. There are proposals to harmonise and standardise the approach across all providers.

Under Monitor's investment regime, for investments considered as 'significant' or 'material' (25% or 10% of turnover respectively), the FT's Board of Directors must sign a statement to say that the affordability of the transaction has been fully considered; the figures are also subject to independent review. All 'significant' transactions must be notified to Monitor.

The key underlying principle for all organisations is that total borrowing must be affordable.

Borrowing, in the context of borrowing limits monitored by the Department of Health, has a wide definition and includes all loans (whatever their source) as well as finance leases including private finance initiative (PFI) schemes (see the next section).

Public dividend capital (PDC)

Before the introduction of loan funding for capital investment, NHS trusts received capital funding allocations. These took the form of public dividend capital (PDC) – a type of long-term government finance. Although new PDC has in effect been replaced with loan funding it is possible that it can be issued to non-foundation trusts and FTs on either an interest or non-interest bearing basis. In some cases, new PDC is issued to assist an NHS body in financial difficulties and in others it is used to allow access to Department of Health capital budgets for specific initiatives (for example, in relation to carbon efficiency).

Where PDC funding has been agreed with the Department of Health for a capital project, then a 'PDC limit' is set (by the Department). This is similar to a cash based capital resource limit. Non-foundation trusts and FTs can only access PDC once all internally generated funds have been used and when the cash is required to pay for the capital project. In other words, cash backed PDC cannot be accessed ('drawn down') in advance of need.

It is worth noting that if an asset is transferred between two NHS trusts, a 'circular flow of funds' is required whereby the asset is paid for with PDC; PDC equivalent to the value of the asset is then removed from the 'seller'. This flow of funds does not involve the transfer of cash between any of the bodies involved.

Public private partnerships

Although there has been a fall in the use of public private partnerships as a result of the economic downturn, they remain an option for delivering capital investment schemes. The main routes are discussed below.

Private finance initiative (PFI)

Traditional PFI schemes have been used for a number of years and involved the creation of partnerships between the public and private sectors, allowing the NHS to raise funds for capital projects from commercial organisations. The financing of the construction of the asset was the responsibility of the PFI provider and the idea was that capital investment was funded without recourse to public money. Private companies were contracted to design and build the assets which were then 'leased back' to the public sector, usually over a period of around 30 years. The contract set out in detail the obligations of each party over the agreed period. The contract usually contained a service element relating to the building – for example, cleaning, catering, security and maintenance.

Private finance 2

Following a review of public private partnerships by the Treasury, a new approach to private sector involvement in public sector infrastructure projects has been developed. Under this approach, the Government acts as a minority equity co-investor with investments managed by a commercially focused central unit located within HM Treasury. Recognising the importance of greater transparency, information will be published in relation to the progress of individual projects as well as the private sector returns generated. An NHS central procurement unit is likely to undertake the procurement role. A preferred bidder will then have responsibility for asset design, construction, maintenance and renewal through the award of a single contract. Greater flexibility is anticipated by excluding 'soft facilities management' from service contracts (for example, catering and cleaning).

Local improvement finance trusts (LIFT)

Local improvement finance trusts (LIFTs) have been used to develop and improve primary care and community-based facilities. Delivered by Community Health Partnerships (CHP – a limited company wholly owned by the Department of Health) on behalf of the Department, a partnership is established with the local health economy through a LIFT company. This is a limited company with the NHS, CHP and the private sector partner as shareholders. The company owns and maintains the building and leases the premises back to the NHS. Prior to April 2013, local primary care trusts were shareholders in the company but their interests have now transferred to CHP with NHS Property Services ltd assuming day-to-day responsibility for running the ex-PCT LIFT estate under a service contract with CHP.

There are a small number of LIFT schemes where a non-foundation trust or FT is the lead lessor and their interests have not transferred to CHP.

Leases

A lease is often considered a suitable alternative to the outright purchase of a capital asset.

A lease is defined as an arrangement between two parties (the 'lessor' and the 'lessee') 'whereby the lessor conveys to the lessee in return for a payment or series of payments the right to use an asset for an agreed period of time'.

There are two types of lease:

- where the lessor transfers to the lessee substantially all the economic benefits and risks of asset ownership. This is referred to as a finance lease
- any lease which is not a finance lease is an operating lease. These are likely to relate to smaller assets and equipment such as cars and photocopiers or parts of larger assets such as a floor of an office block.

The type of lease depends on who bears the risks or benefits from the rewards of using the asset and is assessed using a series of tests set out in international accounting standard 17 (IAS 17). However, land is not normally treated as a finance lease unless it is expected that the title will pass to the lessee at the end of the lease or the lease is very long term (999 years).

Donations and grants

Charitable donations can be an important source of funds to support capital investment but the trustees (usually the NHS corporate body) must ensure that the expenditure is in line with the charitable fund's purpose as set out in its governing documents.

Some NHS bodies also receive grants from bodies such as the Lottery Fund to finance the purchase of capital assets.

Since 2011/12, charitable donations and grants are recognised as income by the NHS body in the year that any conditions attached to the donation are met. When a donation or grant is to be used to buy a capital asset this means that the income is recognised in the year that the asset is purchased. However, the cost of the asset is spread over the life of that asset in the form of depreciation charges which results in a timing difference between the recognition of the income and expenditure.

From 2013/14 the in-year impact of any donations will be included in the accounts of NHS organisations (where the charitable fund is consolidated into the NHS organisation's accounts) but is excluded for the purposes of determining whether or not the organisation has met its financial duties. This is because any donated assets are gifted to the organisation and so do not count as its own expenditure. For more about NHS charitable funds, see chapter 19.

The Cost of Capital

Capital charges

Until 2010/11, all Government bodies had a system of capital charges to recognise and account for the cost of using assets owned by the organisation. Capital charges comprised two elements:

- capital charge – a real cash charge for the cost of capital (similar to debt interest)
- depreciation – a non-cash charge reflecting the cost of using an asset over its useful life.

Capital charges were designed to:

- ensure that there was a consistent approach to applying the cost of capital in the NHS
- provide incentives to use capital efficiently and dispose of surplus assets to generate cash for capital investment
- ensure that the cost of capital was fully reflected in the costing of healthcare services, so that fair comparisons were possible, both within the NHS and between the NHS and the private sector
- promote effective planning for the replacement of capital assets.

In 2010/11, the cost of capital charge was abolished by HM Treasury. However, the Department of Health retained the PDC dividend for trusts and FTs (see below). Commissioning organisations (which do not have PDC) are not subject to capital charges other than depreciation.

PDC dividend

The PDC dividend is derived by applying a percentage 'rate of return' to an organisation's 'average relevant net assets', calculated as follows:

Average Net Relevant Assets Calculation

The average of the organisation's total assets and reserves (i.e. the opening balance at 1st April added to the closing balance at 31st March divided by 2)

Less   the net book value of donated assets and lottery-funded assets held
Less   the cash held in Government Banking Service[4] accounts including any National Loans Fund balances
Plus   the value of any notional income balance that funds a donated asset.

The percentage used is 3.5% for non-foundation trusts and FTs and is payable in two instalments during the year.

Depreciation

Depreciation is calculated annually to reflect the cost of 'using up' the asset during its useful life – a number of assumptions are used:

Depreciation – Assumptions Used

- Land is considered to have an infinite life and is not depreciated
- Buildings, installations and fittings are depreciated over their assessed useful lives, with both the value and life expectancy determined periodically by a qualified valuer
- Assets in the course of construction are not depreciated until they are brought into use
- Equipment is depreciated over its useful economic life
- Leased assets classified as capital are depreciated over the shorter of the lease term remaining or the asset's remaining economic life

---

Depreciation is usually calculated on a 'straight line basis' which means it is assumed that the asset will be 'used up' evenly over its life. As depreciation is calculated on asset values which are subject to revaluation, the depreciation charge and total value of the assets held will vary each year.

Interest

Non-foundation NHS trusts must pay interest on capital investment loans twice a year in addition to the repayment of the loan amount itself. Linked to the National Loans Fund rate, interest payments are largely fixed over the duration of the loan unless the loan is re-financed during that period.

---

[4] The Government Banking Service is the banking shared service provider to Government and the wider public sector. It is responsible for holding the working balances of Government departments and other public bodies in high-level accounts at the Bank of England.

FTs must also pay interest charges on any borrowing including commercial loans. The interest rates on any loans from the FTFF are also linked to the National Loans Fund rate. Commercial loans attract a market rate.

For all NHS organisations, interest is also payable on the balance of outstanding finance leases.

Accounting for Capital

Accounting standards

The Treasury has developed a *Financial Reporting Manual* that sets out how accounting standards should be implemented in the public sector. The Department of Health also produces a *Manual for Accounts* for non-foundation organisations and FTs follow Monitor's *Annual Reporting Manual.* For commissioners, guidance is issued by NHS England. The following accounting standards are of particular relevance when accounting for capital:

- IAS 16 Property, Plant and Equipment
- IAS 17 Leases
- IAS 20 Accounting for Government Grants and Disclosure of Government Assistance
- IFRS 5 Non-current Assets Held for Sale
- IAS 36 Impairment of Assets
- IAS 38 Intangible Assets
- IAS 40 Investment Property
- IFRIC 4 Determining whether an arrangement contains a lease
- IFRIC 12 Service Concession Arrangements.

Purchasing an asset

Where an asset is purchased the accounting entries are:

Debit: Non-current assets: property, plant and equipment/intangible assets
Credit: Cash

Valuation

On acquisition, capital assets are recorded at their 'fair value' – the market value for their existing use. Specialised property such as hospitals for which a market value cannot be easily determined, is valued at the cost of replacing it with an equivalent, modern one, not an exact replica of what currently exists. This is the 'depreciated replacement cost' approach, also known as the 'modern equivalent asset basis'.

Under IAS 16, organisations must consider whether the recorded value of their tangible assets continues to reflect fair value taking into account market volatility. For example, if the local property market is particularly volatile or the organisation embarks upon a significant capital expenditure project, annual revaluations may be needed to keep the recorded value up to date. When an individual asset (for example, a piece of medical equipment) is revalued, all assets of its type must also be revalued. In the absence of a significant change, revaluation may be needed less frequently.

Each year, an assessment must be made of whether the valuations are materially correct or not. This will involve consideration of the volatility of the property market and usually requires discussion with a professional valuer. In years where a professional valuation has not been undertaken, the value given to land and buildings will need to be reviewed and any changes appropriately evidenced to support the preparation of the accounts. Valuation is also required when:

- organisations merge
- there is a major change in use
- an asset formerly under construction is brought into use.

Most intangible assets (i.e. assets that have a financial value even though they are not visible – for example, goodwill) are recorded at cost less 'amortisation' (equivalent to depreciation but for intangible assets) as a proxy for fair value. However, where a market value is readily available then this should be used.

Gains

Gains in asset value may occur following a revaluation by an external reviewer or, for equipment assets, by a review undertaken by the finance and/or estates departments to provide a new fair value. To account for a gain, the entries needed are as follows:

Debit: Non-current assets

Credit: Revaluation reserve

Losses (including impairments)

Impairments occur where there is a loss in the value of a non-current asset (i.e. assets that cannot be converted to cash in less than a year) compared to its recorded value. This can be due to:

- a loss of economic benefit to an asset itself – for example, it is physically damaged
- the asset becoming surplus to requirements
- a change in the asset or its environment which has permanently reduced its capacity to generate revenue.

IAS 36 is relevant here. However, HM Treasury guidance diverges from IAS 36 and requires organisations to identify the cause of impairment as the result of either:

- the consumption of economic benefits or service potential **OR**
- a loss following revaluation.

In the first scenario, the resulting loss is charged to operating expenses as follows:

> Debit: Operating expenses
> Credit: Non-current assets

However, where there has been a previous upward revaluation for the asset and a revaluation reserve balance exists, a transfer is made from the revaluation reserve to the general fund/ retained earnings:

> Debit: Revaluation reserve (with the lower of the total impairment or the revaluation reserve balance for that asset)
> Credit: General fund/retained earnings

In the event of a revaluation loss, the reduction should initially be charged to the revaluation reserve to the extent that a balance exists for the asset. Any remaining amount is charged to operating expenses:

> Debit: Revaluation reserve (up to the value of the corresponding revaluation reserve balance for the asset) and/or
> Debit: Operating expenses (if there are insufficient funds within the revaluation reserve to fund the impairment)
> Credit: Non-current assets

If impaired assets then have an upward valuation, the charge made to expenditure can be reversed to the extent that the upward revaluation reverses the original impairment. It is therefore important to record all impairment charges by individual asset to enable entries to be reversed if needed.

Accounting for the sale or disposal of an asset

The accounting entries needed for sale or disposal are as follows:

Profit on sale or disposal

> Debit: Cash
> Credit: Non-current assets – to the value of the asset held
> Credit: Other operating income – with the profit element

Loss on sale or disposal

> Debit: Cash
> Debit: Operating expenses – with the loss element
> Credit: Non-current assets – to the value of the asset held

Leases

The two types of lease are accounted for as follows:

- finance leases: the asset is recorded in the asset register with a corresponding lease liability. The asset is treated as if it had been bought outright as soon as it becomes operational. It forms part of average relevant net assets for PDC dividend calculations, is subject to depreciation and is revalued in the same way as any owned asset. The lease liability is written down as the capital element is repaid
- operating leases: rental payments are treated as operating expenditure.

Leases are a complex area in accounting terms and are covered by IAS 17. Other relevant standards that need to be considered are IFRIC 4 (*Determining Whether an Arrangement Contains a Lease*) and IFRIC 12 (*Service Concession Arrangements*).

PFI and LIFT schemes

PFI and LIFT schemes are also complicated arrangements to account for. Relevant accounting standards that need to be considered are IFRIC 12 (*Service Concession Arrangements*) and SIC 29 (*Service Concession Arrangements: Disclosures*).

Key Components in Accounting for PFI and LIFT Schemes

- Organisations must consider whether the scheme represents a service concession under IFRIC 12 for which a number of specific 'tests' exist, and if not, whether the scheme is a finance lease or an operating lease
- The asset is recognised in the organisation's accounts at 'fair value' – the capital cost of the asset at the inception of the scheme which is determined using the contractor's financial model
- A finance lease liability is shown equal to the fair value of the asset
- The unitary payment (i.e. the payment made by the public sector organisation to its private sector partner) is allocated between:
  - payment for services
  - payment for the property:
    - repayment of the liability
    - interest charge relating to the lease
    - contingent rent (this is a rent which is not fixed throughout the contract – it usually varies in relation to RPI or a percentage of RPI over the life of the contract)
  - life cycle costs relating to future capital expenditure.
- Depreciation and other changes in value must be accounted for as with any other asset owned by the organisation

Donated assets

Assets funded by donation require specific identification in the asset register. The most common method of receiving a donated asset is for it to be purchased by the NHS organisation and for an invoice to be raised to the charitable body funding the asset; this can help with identification. It is worth noting that donated assets do not form part of the PDC dividend calculation. Donated assets are accounted for as follows:

> Debit: Non-current assets
> Credit: Cash
> Debit: Cash
> Credit: Donated income

Income will fluctuate in line with the receipt of new donated assets, either improving or worsening the revenue position according to whether more or less donated income is received as compared to the depreciation charge on the overall value of donated assets.

Key Learning Points

- Capital assets deliver a benefit to an organisation over a period of time
- Capital assets can be tangible or intangible
- In order to account appropriately for capital assets, a detailed asset register must be maintained and kept up to date
- Organisations work within a system of controls and financial limits to ensure that taxpayers' money used to finance capital expenditure is safeguarded
- It is important to consider capital needs and plan to meet them; organisations must consider the affordability of financing capital investment as well as the on-going revenue costs within the context of the capital controls
- A well-structured, logical and concise business case can help explain the case for capital investment. It may be subject to external approval depending on its value
- The potential sources of funding for capital investments vary by type of NHS organisation – not every option is available to every type of organisation
- Commissioners are not expected to hold many capital assets. Ex-primary care trust property has been transferred to NHS Property Services Ltd and LIFT schemes to Community Health Partnerships Ltd
- Commissioners have limited access to sources of capital funding
- Non-foundation trusts and FTs have access to a number of sources of capital funding: internally generated resources; borrowing; public/private partnerships; leases, grants and donations. NHS organisations may also have access to public dividend capital (PDC) in certain circumstances
- A cost of capital charge is incurred either as PDC dividend or interest payments; depreciation is also charged.

References and Further Reading

Manual for Accounts, Department of Health (FINMAN website): www.info.doh.gov.uk/doh/finman.nsf/

NHS Property Services Ltd: www.property.nhs.uk/

Community Health Partnerships (including LIFT): www.communityhealthpartnerships.co.uk/

Health and Social Care Act 2012: www.legislation.gov.uk/ukpga/2012/7/contents/enacted

Risk Assessment Framework, Monitor, 2013:
www.monitor-nhsft.gov.uk/home/news-events-and-publications/our-publications

Delivering High Quality Care for Patients: The Accountability Framework for NHS Trust Boards, NHS TDA, 2013:
www.ntda.nhs.uk/wp-content/uploads/2012/04/framework_050413_web.pdf

National Loans Fund rates – available via: www.dmo.gov.uk/index.aspx?page=PWLB/NLF_Rates

Public Private Partnerships guidance, HM Treasury:
www.hm-treasury.gov.uk/infrastructure_public_private_partnerships.htm

Private Finance 2 (PF2), HM Treasury:
www.hm-treasury.gov.uk/infrastructure_pfireform.htm

Accounting for PFI under IFRS and Accounting for NHS LIFT under IFRS, Department of Health, 2009: www.info.doh.gov.uk/doh/finman.nsf/4db79df91d978b6c00256728004f9d6b/
5c86c759beddaecf80257654003623c5?OpenDocument

Budgeting for PFI and LIFT and ESA 95: www.info.doh.gov.uk/doh/finman.nsf/
4db79df91d978b6c00256728004f9d6b/a4e263b8ca7ef596802576a90038a6f8?OpenDocument

International Accounting Standards: www.ifrs.org/IFRSs/Pages/IAS.aspx

International Financial Reporting Standards Interpretations (IFRICs):
www.ifrs.org/IFRSs/Pages/IFRICs.aspx

Guidance on asset valuation, HM Treasury:
www.hm-treasury.gov.uk/d/guidance_on_asset_valuation.pdf

Government Financial Reporting Manual, Treasury: www.hm-treasury.gov.uk/frem_index.htm

Annual Reporting Manual, Monitor, 2013: www.monitor-nhsft.gov.uk/home/news-events-and-publications/our-publications/browse-category/guidance-foundation-trusts/mandat-5

Chapter 16: Commissioning

> **Overview**
>
> This chapter explains what commissioning, what it aims to achieve and what it involves in practice. In particular it works through the 'commissioning cycle' and explains what each step involves.

What is Commissioning?

The Department of Health has described commissioning as 'the process of ensuring that the health and care services provided effectively meet the needs of the population. It is a complex process with responsibilities ranging from assessing population needs, prioritising health outcomes, procuring products and services, and managing service providers'. However, what it boils down to in practice is commissioners negotiating agreements with service providers (in the NHS, private and voluntary sectors) to meet the health needs of a particular population.

Although commissioning has existed since the start of the NHS, reforms introduced by the Labour Government to the financial regime and in particular the introduction of payment by results, practice based commissioning and the world class commissioning initiative made it more prominent.

> **Payment by Results** (PbR) is the funding system for some of the care provided to NHS patients in England and applies to most (but not all) acute services. Hospitals are paid a nationally set price or tariff for the work they do and commissioning negotiations for these activities focus on quality and volume rather than price. For services that are **not** covered by payment by results, prices are negotiated by the host commissioner along with quality and volume. See chapter 18 for more about PbR and how NHS services are paid for.
>
> **Practice Based Commissioning** (PBC) was introduced in 2005/06 based on the assumption that primary care professionals were in the best position to decide what services their patients needed and to redesign them accordingly. Under PBC, responsibility for commissioning along with an associated notional budget from the primary care trust (PCT) was allocated to some primary care clinicians. The budget was notional because the PCT remained legally responsible for managing the money and negotiating and managing all contracts with providers.
>
> **World Class Commissioning** was introduced in 2007 and comprised four main elements (a vision; a set of organisational competencies; an annual assurance system that reviewed PCTs' progress and a support and development framework). WCC emphasised the importance of getting commissioning right and saw it as being at the heart of delivering an NHS that is 'fair, personalised, effective and safe, and which is focused relentlessly on improving the quality of care'.

The Coalition Government has also recognised the importance of getting commissioning right with a new structure that includes NHS England and GP led clinical commissioning groups (CCGs). This new approach places primary care clinicians at the heart of the commissioning process with CCGs fully accountable for managing the funding they receive from NHS England and negotiating contracts with providers of services.

The Aims of Commissioning

Although the key players in the commissioning field have changed, the function itself continues with the same overall objectives. The focus for NHS commissioners and the 'organising principle' that underlies all that they do is quality. This means that the overarching goals for commissioning are to achieve:

- improved health outcomes
- reduced health inequalities
- improved provider quality
- increased productivity.

However, in practice commissioners are constrained by the fact that demand for healthcare always exceeds the level of funds available and so there is a need for them to make choices and to prioritise. This involves a focus on local needs, targets and desired outcomes together with reviewing services in the search for greater effectiveness, economy and efficiency. NHS commissioners are also expected to achieve improvements in relation to the five domains set out in the *NHS Outcomes Framework* and follow planning guidance issued each year by NHS England.

NHS Outcomes Framework Domains

Domain 1   Preventing people from dying prematurely.
Domain 2   Enhancing quality of life for people with long-term conditions.
Domain 3   Helping people to recover from episodes of ill health or following injury.
Domain 4   Ensuring that people have a positive experience of care.
Domain 5   Treating and caring for people in a safe environment; and protecting them from avoidable harm.

Another source of information available to commissioners that is worth mentioning at this point is the *Clinical Commissioning Group Outcomes Indicator Set* developed by The National Institute for Health and Care Excellence (NICE) and published by NHS England. This is designed to help commissioners by providing comparative information about the quality of health services commissioned and health outcomes achieved (i.e. it does not look at the commissioning process but at the services commissioned). The *Indicator Set* contains indicators from the *NHS Outcomes Framework* that can be broken down to CCG level and other additional indicators – for example linked to NICE quality standards. Each year, NHS England's planning guidance includes details of relevant indicators for the forthcoming year.

The Commissioning Cycle

Commissioning does not follow a pre-set template and cannot be done once and forgotten about – rather it is a continuous process with many different elements. It is only by going through the entire process – often referred to as 'the commissioning cycle' – that a realistic commissioning plan can be drawn up and an associated budget developed. This cycle is shown below in diagrammatic form:[1]

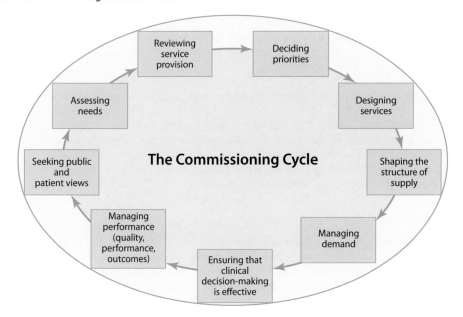

The Commissioning Cycle

- Reviewing service provision
- Deciding priorities
- Designing services
- Shaping the structure of supply
- Managing demand
- Ensuring that clinical decision-making is effective
- Managing performance (quality, performance, outcomes)
- Seeking public and patient views
- Assessing needs

These activities are usually grouped into three key phases – planning, procurement and managing/monitoring.

Planning

Assessing health needs with a focus on patient outcomes

Assessing needs involves planning ahead so that an organisation knows what services are required to meet the needs of the population served. This cannot be done in isolation – commissioners must work with others (for example, public health professionals, local authority Health and Wellbeing Boards (HWBs), patients and the local community) to gather the information they need.

In looking at needs, it is important that the focus is on commissioning services that will result in good patient outcomes rather than the more traditional emphasis on processes. For example, the test of effective commissioning for knee operations could be whether or not patients can return to work or drive again rather than the number of operations that are carried out over a set period of time. As we will see later, this outcomes focus involves thinking

---

[1] Adapted from a version that appeared in the Department of Health's 2006 guidance *Health Reform in England: update and commissioning framework*.

about developing new and innovative ways of contracting which incentivises providers to deliver the desired outcomes.

Reviewing service provision and identifying gaps or areas where change is needed

This stage involves using the local Joint Strategic Needs Assessment (JSNA) and the Joint Health and Wellbeing Strategy (JHWS) – both led by the HWB established by the local authority (see chapter 8). It also involves:

- looking at outcomes from services – in other words, are services delivering what they should?
- using benchmarking data – for example, from NHS RightCare's *Atlas of Variation*
- reviewing the latest guidance and assessing its impact – for example, from NICE
- analysing feedback from service users
- being aware of any guidance or recommendations that inspectors or regulators have issued – for example, CQC and Monitor.

Deciding priorities

This is a tricky area as it involves commissioners taking tough decisions about exactly how to spend the limited pot of money that they have available. Inevitably, not all needs can be met and so relative priorities must be established in a logical and objective way. Commissioners need to link these decisions to their overall objectives, plans and budgets. They must also take account of patient choice and the views of the local community and other partners. Another consideration is the need for openness and transparency in the approach to deciding priorities so that everyone can understand why decisions are made and see that the approach is objective and impartial.

Procurement

Once planning has been carried out, the next stage is for commissioners to buy or 'procure' the services that they have decided are needed whilst bearing in mind the need to provide for both competition and patient choice.

Designing services

The first step in this process is to ensure that the way services are designed is in line with the agreed priorities. This may involve reshaping the way things are delivered in consultation with GP practices and other providers. This is where NHS England's commissioning guidelines and model care pathways fit in.

Shaping the structure of supply

Once commissioners are clear about what it is they want to buy they need to make sure this is specified clearly so that service providers know exactly what they are expected to deliver. In some instances, commissioners may also need to encourage changes in provision to meet their requirements – for example, so that services are provided closer to home or in different ways or to fill gaps in the range of services provided. This involves working with local authorities and potential service providers to:

- develop service specifications
- understand any barriers that might prevent potential providers from coming forward and (in some cases and where it is appropriate) addressing them
- identify incentives that could stimulate supply – for example, using 3 year contracts that recognise that the level of work will increase gradually.

Managing demand whilst ensuring appropriate access to care

Managing demand is one of the most challenging aspects of commissioning as the care and services that patients need during the year must be matched with contracts that are agreed in advance. Effective demand management is therefore inextricably linked to shaping the supply of services and ensuring that the services that are available are clinically appropriate. It also involves reducing clinical variation in referrals made by GPs and in consultants' clinical practice.

In practical terms managing demand means that commissioners must:

- have access to reliable, timely activity monitoring information – for example, in relation to referral patterns
- anticipate in-year changes – for example in screening programmes; care pathways; new providers; NICE guidance
- have in place activity management plans
- identify and follow best practice
- ensure that enough resources are devoted to health promotion and education, preventative measures and communication.

Increasingly, commissioners also need to look beyond the costs of individual treatments that may be needed during a year to consider the likely total cost of patient care across several years (this may include social care costs). There are a number of tools and techniques that commissioners can use to 'join up' the information they need to be able to assess future demand in this way – for example:

- risk stratification – to identify patients with long term conditions who may need closer management or those who use hospital services regularly and are more likely to have re-admissions
- predictive modelling – by identifying the probability of future events occurring to groups of patients, interventions can be planned and executed.

With their detailed knowledge of patients' needs, GPs are at the forefront of demand management, specifying services and developing new care pathways. They can also influence how their patients behave – for example, by encouraging self-care and preventative measures and by educating them about which services should be accessed when (for example, when to use pharmacy services rather than minor injuries units). This can help reduce the number of referrals and improve the overall quality of patient care.

Contracting

Although 'contracting' does not appear on its own in the commissioning cycle diagram it is a key stage in the procurement phase. Unlike other sectors of the economy, the NHS uses a standard contract for the commissioning of all NHS clinical services (except primary care[2]). This contract can be adapted to suit a broad range of services and delivery models – in other words the standard contract provides a framework that can then be added to locally.

The healthcare services that are covered by the contract may be provided by non-foundation and foundation trusts or other public or private sector providers (i.e. by 'any qualified provider'). Contracts must be signed before the start of the financial year with any disputes resolved swiftly. Any outstanding problems are dealt with via mediation and formal adjudication.

Commissioners must enforce the standard terms of the contract. These include penalties for under-performance and requirements such as a duty of openness and the need for a 'friends and family test' to be offered to all patients in acute inpatient hospital wards and accident and emergency departments.

For services covered by PbR, the standard contract uses the nationally set price or tariff. For services that fall outside the scope of PbR the standard contract must still be followed with details of whatever payment system applies entered. There are three main 'non-PbR' options for agreeing payments – block; cost and volume and cost per case.

Payment options for non PbR activity

Block payments (or 'block contracts') – this approach is used most notably for community healthcare services where a unit of healthcare may not easily be determined. Under a block contract, commissioners effectively pay healthcare providers a fixed amount of money for access to a defined range and volume of service for the year ahead. The provider receives an amount of funding irrespective of the number of patients treated or the type of treatment provided.

Cost and volume – here a fixed sum is paid for access to a defined range and volume of services but if there is a variation from the intended level of activity, there is a variation in payment levels according to a 'variation', or 'threshold agreement' clause.

Cost per case – this approach is most commonly used for procedures that are infrequent, unpredictable, or can have significant cost variations. They are also used for individual, expensive, and bespoke care package agreements (for example, the placement of patients in medium secure mental health facilities).

---

[2] The standard contract is not used for primary care services provided by GPs, dentists, opticians and community pharmacists as these are governed by separate contracts and form part of NHS England's direct commissioning activities – see chapters 4 and 6 for more details.

NHS England is responsible for reviewing and updating the standard contract documentation. Details are available on its website.

See chapter 18 for more about PbR and how NHS services are paid for.

In letting contracts, commissioners must also consider how and when to introduce competition to improve services. The Department of Health made clear when announcing new regulations on choice and competition in March 2013, that there 'is no requirement to put all contracts out to competitive tender' and that 'Monitor has no power to force the competitive tendering of services'. To help commissioners in this area NHS England and Monitor are developing a 'choice and competition website'.

Managing and monitoring

Ensuring effective clinical decision-making

Although contracts are agreed by NHS England or CCGs, each referral that a primary care clinician (usually a GP) makes is effectively a mini commissioning decision that commits money. Those making these decisions therefore need to:

- recognise the broader context
- be aware of service options
- be able to justify their decisions
- accept peer review of performance
- understand the implications of their decisions.

Managing performance

Commissioners need to ensure that the services they have bought are delivered in line with the specifications they set out in their contracts in terms of quantity, quality and price. They must also review performance in relation to:

- **achieving national standards** – for example, the NHS Constitution 18 week waiting time and patients not having an urgent operation cancelled twice. NHS England expects commissioners to 'use their contracting muscle' to penalise such failings
- **quality** – contracts between commissioners and providers allow for a proportion of providers' income to be conditional on quality, innovation and the achievement of local quality improvement goals. At present, this payment framework (known as 'Commissioning for Quality and Innovation' or CQUIN) allows providers to earn up to 2.5% 'on top of actual outturn value' for all standard contracts (2% is determined locally and 0.5% is linked to national goals where they apply). Guidance on CQUIN is available on NHS England's website which explains the rationale for the approach and sets out in broad terms what a CQUIN scheme should look like. In particular, the guidance emphasises that although the detailed content of a scheme is 'for local discretion and discussion between the commissioner and provider' they must cover safety; effectiveness (including clinical outcomes and 'patient reported outcomes'); user experience (including timeliness of provision) and innovation

- **never events** – there is a national set of 'never events' that must be included as part of contract agreements with providers. Any such events must be reported to the Care Quality Commission via the National Reporting and Learning Service. Department of Health guidance requires commissioners to withhold payment for an episode of care in which a never event occurs, as well as for subsequent treatment of the consequences of a never event. The full list is included within the standard contract documentation – examples include wrong site surgery; retained instrument post operation; wrong route of administration of chemotherapy and inpatient suicide by non-collapsible rails
- complaints/patient survey data
- key performance indicators
- outcomes in specifications
- activity management (for example, via referral analysis).

Undertaking patient and public feedback

Every CCG has a duty to prepare a commissioning plan before the start of each year that shows how it intends to use its budget and improve outcomes for patients. As mentioned earlier, these plans are discussed with the relevant HWB to ensure that they reflect the JSNA and JHWS. CCGs (and NHS England) are also under a duty to ensure that people who receive services 'are involved in its planning and development, and to promote and extend public and patient involvement and choice.' This means making use of patient satisfaction surveys and using these to inform the next commissioning round. To ensure that this information is available, the requirement for patient feedback is often built into service specifications.

Effective Commissioning

To be effective commissioners need to:

- have the necessary skills and experience (either themselves or via commissioning support units hosted by NHS England – see chapter 4)
- engage with a broad range of clinicians
- improve community engagement
- ensure choice for patients.

They must also have access to information and skills that will support their decisions. To help them in this area, a national information system known as the 'secondary uses service' (SUS) collects patient level activity information from providers and makes it available to commissioners. This system then applies the tariff to providers' activity information, calculates the payment due and notifies each commissioner. Other important sources of information include:

- programme budgeting – information on how resources are spent across 23 different programmes of care is collected from all commissioners and allows CCGs to benchmark their own spend in a particular area with that of a similar organisation covering a similar population (see chapter 10)
- population risk assessments
- historical referral patterns

- details of past spending patterns and how this compares (for example, with other GP practices)
- real time information to monitor actual activity against plans and expenditure against budgets.

Who are the Commissioners in the NHS and how do they approach their Responsibilities?

The key commissioners in the NHS are NHS England and clinical commissioning groups (CCGs). Local authorities are also involved as they are responsible for health improvement and public health spending. These organisations' structures, accountabilities and roles are described in chapters 4, 5 and 8 but it is worth noting here that they can use a number of different approaches – for example:

- NHS England commissions some services – see chapter 4
- CCGs commission services themselves – see chapter 5
- where it makes sense for the health economy as whole (for example, to achieve economies of scale), CCGs work together collaboratively. This may mean using a lead commissioner approach where a single contract is negotiated by the lead commissioner with the local service provider and it is managed across all member CCGs. NHS England has produced a model collaborative commissioning agreement for CCGs to use when working together in this way
- network arrangements (for example, for cancer services) may undertake some commissioning functions on behalf of their constituent CCGs
- partnership working with local authorities. Since April 2013, local authorities have been responsible for public health activities and lead on health improvement and reducing health inequalities. They also jointly commission some services with CCGs (see chapter 8).

Key Learning Points

- Commissioners negotiate agreements with service providers to meet the health needs of their population
- The aim is to improve health outcomes, reduce health inequalities, improve provider quality and increase productivity
- Commissioners have to make tough choices as demand for healthcare services always exceeds the level of funds available
- Commissioning is a continuous process with many different elements grouped under three phases – planning, procurement and managing/monitoring
- There is a standard NHS contract used for the commissioning of all NHS clinical services (except primary care). Where PbR applies, the prices used are dictated by the national the tariff
- For services not covered by PbR, the standard contract must still be followed with details of the relevant payment system entered – there are three main options: block; cost and volume and cost per case
- Commissioners must ensure national standards (for example, as set out in the NHS Constitution) are met and penalise any failings
- Contracts allow for a proportion of providers' income to depend on quality – the CQUIN payment framework is used to achieve this

- 'Never events' must be included as part of the contract agreements. When they occur they must be reported to the Care Quality Commission via the National Reporting and Learning Service
- The key players in the commissioning field are NHS England, CCGs and local authorities.

References and Further Reading

The NHS Outcomes Framework 2013/14, NHS England:
www.gov.uk/government/publications/nhs-outcomes-framework-2013-to-2014

Health Reform in England: update and commissioning framework, Department of Health, 2006 (archived web pages): http://webarchive.nationalarchives.gov.uk/20080814090418/dh.gov.uk/en/Publicationsandstatistics/Publications/PublicationsPolicyAndGuidance/DH_4137226

Information about the Clinical Commissioning Group Outcome Indicator Set, NICE, 2013:
www.nice.org.uk/aboutnice/ccgois/CCGOIS.jsp#X-201301091452371

Clinical Commissioning Group Outcome Indicator Set, NHS England, 2013:
www.england.nhs.uk/ccg-ois/

Information about predictive modelling:
www.connectingforhealth.nhs.uk/systemsandservices/qipp/library/predictivefs.pdf

NHS Atlas of Variation in Healthcare Services, NHS RightCare:
www.rightcare.nhs.uk/index.php/nhs-atlas/

NHS Standard Contract 2013/14, NHS England: www.england.nhs.uk/nhs-standard-contract/

Information about choice and competition in procurement, NHS England:
www.england.nhs.uk/2013/03/19/choice-competition/

Regulations on healthcare procurement, patient choice and competition, March 2013:
https://www.gov.uk/government/publications/regulations-on-healthcare-procurement-patient-choice-and-competition-laid

Everyone Counts: Planning for Patients 2013/14, NHS England, 2012:
www.england.nhs.uk/everyonecounts/

NHS Friends and Family Test guidance, Department of Health, 2013: https://www.gov.uk/government/publications/nhs-friends-and-family-test-guidance-on-scoring-and-presenting-results-published

Commissioning for Quality and Innovation (CQUIN) 2013/14, NHS England, 2013:
www.england.nhs.uk/everyonecounts/

The Never Events Policy Framework: an update to the never events policy, Department of Health, 2012: https://www.gov.uk/government/uploads/system/uploads/attachment_data/file/127087/never-events-policy-framework-update-to-policy.pdf.pdf

National Reporting and Learning Service: www.nrls.npsa.nhs.uk/report-a-patient-safety-incident/about-reporting-patient-safety-incidents/

Secondary Uses Service (SUS): www.hscic.gov.uk/sus

Model Collaborative Commissioning Agreement for CCGs, NHS England, 2013 – under CCG development on the CCG resources page: www.england.nhs.uk/resources/resources-for-ccgs/

Chapter 17: Costing

Overview

This chapter looks at an activity that is increasingly prominent in today's NHS. Although costing has always been important, the use of payment by results (PbR) for most acute hospital activity (and its introduction into mental health services) means that the production of accurate cost information by NHS organisations is critical as it informs the development of the national tariff. Within a context of limited growth and the need to deliver efficiencies, NHS organisations must have a detailed understanding of their own cost base so that they can manage their activities effectively within the available resources whilst delivering higher quality care and better value.

What is Costing?

Costing is the quantification, in financial terms, of the value of resources consumed in carrying out a particular activity or producing a certain unit of output. Costing therefore involves:

- being clear about the activity whose costs you are seeking to identify – it must be defined clearly and unambiguously
- making sure that the correct costs of everything and everyone involved in carrying out that activity are included in the costing calculation.

It is also important to analyse the costs themselves, how they are related to what is being costed and how they behave.

We will look in more detail at these cost classifications later on in this chapter.

What is Costing Information used for?

In the NHS, costing involves looking closely at healthcare services and identifying how much they cost. This can be at a variety of levels – for example, the total annual cost of the orthopaedic department in a hospital; the cost of a particular activity or group of procedures within that department (for instance, hip replacements) or the cost of treating an individual patient undergoing a hip replacement.

It is important to recognise that costing is not an end in itself – it is only worth doing if the information generated is used in a meaningful way to deliver improvements in healthcare services. In the NHS, costing information is used both within organisations and at a national level.

NHS organisations need costing information for a variety of reasons – for example to:

- help run their businesses effectively and efficiently
- help decision makers, managers and budget holders decide how services should develop in the future

- manage 'services lines' – this involves looking in detail at the income and costs of an organisation's services in much the same way as a private sector company analyses its business units. In practice, this means that the focus is on profitability information (or the contribution made) by specialty. The information gleaned from service line reporting (SLR) is used to 'manage' each service line (hence 'service line management' or SLM) and develop business plans with the organisation overall effectively managed as 'a portfolio of autonomous and accountable business units'
- understand how the costs of providing a particular activity compare with the income received for undertaking that activity
- identify the costs of different activities at different levels (for example, for a particular specialty/department or for an individual patient)
- support the development of commissioning strategies
- compare potential investment opportunities
- build up realistic budgets and plans
- monitor performance and benchmark services
- support negotiations for funding and the agreement of local prices.

At a national level, costing information provided by NHS bodies is used in a variety of ways including to develop:

- healthcare resource groups (HRGs)
- reference cost comparisons
- the tariff for activities covered by PbR
- programme budgeting data which provides information about how NHS money is spent across 23 broad healthcare headings (see chapter 10).

Unless the underlying costing data supplied by health organisations is accurate and collected on a consistent basis, the resulting information (for example, the prices set by Monitor and NHS England for patient funded services under PbR) will not themselves reflect reality or be meaningful. For this reason, Monitor has issued *Approved Costing Guidance* that sets out a recommended approach for all NHS providers covering:

- costing principles
- costing standards
- guidance for reference cost collection
- guidance for the collection of patient-level information and costing systems (PLICS) data.

This guidance also explains the approach to costing and cost collection that should be followed and sets out what service providers will need to do in this area to meet their licence conditions.

Costing Principles

The overriding principle for costing in the NHS is that all costs must be 'fully absorbed'. In other words, every cost (whatever its nature) must be attributed to an activity.

Monitor's guidance also sets out six principles that should be used for all costing exercises.

Monitor's Six Principles

1. Stakeholder engagement – involving all stakeholders, not just finance.
2. Consistency – across and within organisations.
3. Data accuracy – given that multiple data sources are used.
4. Materiality.
5. Causality and objectivity – costing should be based on the accurate assignment of costs with minimum subjectivity.
6. Transparency.

The guidance also recommends that an activity based approach (ABC) to costing is used – this involves identifying activities and their related costs in a structured and logical way. The guidance gives detailed practical guidance for each of six ABC steps that should be followed sequentially.

The Six ABC Steps

1. Define the 'cost object '(i.e. what needs to be costed). This can be a product or service as decided by the provider (for example, an episode of care or service line) OR be specified in guidance (for example, for reference costs, it can be the HRG by episode or spell, outpatient attendance or care cluster in mental health services). We will look at reference costs and HRGs later in this chapter.
2. Identify the activities that are associated with the cost object – for example, by using 'activity and resource input maps' to break down a cost object into the underlying processes, activities and resources used.
3. Establish the relevant costs of those activities.
4. Analyse the costs (see cost classifications below).
5. Assign the costs either via 'tracing', 'cause and effect assignment' or allocation.
6. Validate the output to ensure that cost information is accurate – for example, by sense checking results and benchmarking to confirm that they are reasonable.

Cost Classifications

Monitor's guidance gives details for each step in the ABC process but because it is an area that can cause confusion we are going to look more closely at step 4. This recommends that costs should be categorised using two types of classification namely whether a cost is:

- direct, indirect or an overhead – used to look at how costs relate to what is being costed (i.e. the cost object)
- fixed, semi-fixed or variable – used to look at cost behaviour and 'controllability'.

Direct costs

Direct costs are those costs that relate directly to the particular patient, activity or output being measured and are 'driven' by it. So in the NHS, direct costs are defined in Monitor's guidance as those that 'relate directly to the delivery of patient care. These costs can be directly linked to the delivery of patient care and costs are caused/arise as a result of individual patient episodes of care.' For example, within a hospital ward the cost of drugs supplied and consumed can be directly attributed to that ward by the pharmacy system. Hence, drugs would be a direct cost of the ward.

Indirect costs

Indirect costs cannot be directly attributed to a particular patient or ward but can be indirectly related to them. Such costs are usually collected at an aggregate level and are then allocated to individual cost centres. Generally this is achieved through apportioning the costs using a unit of activity or work measure appropriate to the area concerned. For example, where linen costs cannot be directly attributed to wards these may be allocated using occupied bed days.

The costing guidance defines indirect costs as being 'indirectly related to the delivery of patient care, but cannot always be specifically identified to individual patients. These costs can usually be allocated on an activity basis to service costs.'

Overheads

Overhead costs are defined in the guidance as 'the costs of support services that contribute to the effective running of an NHS provider. These costs cannot be traced or easily attributed to patients and need to be allocated via an appropriate cost driver'. For example, the total heating costs of a hospital may be apportioned to individual departments using floor area or cubic capacity; the costs of finance or human resources may be spread across all cost centres in proportion to those cost centres' total direct and indirect costs. The key here is that overheads are apportioned on a logical and consistent basis.

Fixed costs

Fixed costs are costs that do not change as activity changes over a 12-month period – for example, depreciation.

Semi-fixed costs

Semi-fixed costs are fixed for a given level of activity but change in steps, when activity levels exceed or fall below these given levels. In other words, semi-fixed costs do not move with activity changes on a small scale, but 'jump' or 'step up' when a certain threshold is reached – for example, nursing staff.

Variable costs

Variable costs vary proportionately with changes in activity. In other words, they are directly affected by the number of patients treated or seen – for example, drugs and consumables costs.

Clinical Costing Standards

A key development in the costing arena is the development of clinical costing standards for acute and mental healthcare. These standards have been developed by the HFMA since

2011/12 and are designed to support a bottom-up approach to costing, setting out recommended best practice in producing patient level costs. The acute standards form the second chapter of Monitor's *Approved Costing Guidance*. The mental health costing standards are currently published separately but may be incorporated into the *Approved Costing Guidance* in the future.

Using a more granular approach to costing supports the improved analysis of costs at higher levels (for example, HRGs), but enables organisations to drill down into this data to understand exactly how costs have been incurred. This provides opportunities to improve pathways for patients and identify potential areas for reducing costs.

The costing standards contain ten separate standards to support the classification of costs, identification of 'cost pool groups', allocation of costs, analysis of the total quantum of cost and the underpinning data requirements. The standards also deal with how to manage patient activity which spans the financial year and the need for robust assurance processes.

A materiality and quality score (MAQS) has been developed, and is now included within the costing standards. This score provides a measure of the quality of an organisation's costing processes and data.

Reference Costs and HRGs

Reference costs record activity levels, unit cost data and average length of stay for a range of specified activities and are collected each year from all providers of health services (acute, community and paramedic) to NHS patients using NHS resources. Originally, reference costs were intended for management information purposes but now also form the basis of the PbR tariff.

As there is such a vast range of specific interventions, procedures and diagnoses (around 26,000 patient treatment codes exist), it is not possible to have a separate reference cost (and subsequently, tariff) for each. Instead, a 'currency' is used to collate them into common groupings for the reference cost collection and tariff.

In England the chosen currency is healthcare resource groups or HRGs. HRGs place patient procedures and/or diagnoses into bands, which are 'resource homogenous', that is, clinically similar and consuming similar levels of resources. HRGs 'sit' between top-level specialties and individual patient procedures and treatments, thus reducing the number of individual care profiles that need to be costed. One of the key aims of HRGs is to provide a practical currency to enable sensible discussions between clinicians and managers about the costs of delivering healthcare – it is therefore essential that HRGs are clinically meaningful.

Since 2006/07 'HRG version 4' has been used for costing in the NHS – this comprises more than 1,500 groupings arranged into 21 'chapters' each covering a body system such as the nervous system or cardiac surgery.

HRG 4 is used as the currency for the reference cost collection and admitted patient care is recorded at both finished consultant episode (FCE) and 'spell' level (a spell is the time from entry to discharge – it is used as the basic denominator for PbR as a patient can pass from one consultant to another during a hospital stay).

The submission of reference costs (to the Department of Health for 2012/13 and Monitor thereafter) is mandatory for all NHS providers of services. The guidance underpinning the reference cost collection forms chapter 3 of Monitor's *Approved Costing Guidance*. The information submitted is collated and published annually as the national schedule of reference costs (NSRC). This shows the national average cost for a range of treatments and procedures and can be used by organisations for comparative purposes.

In addition to the NSRC, a national reference cost index (RCI or NRCI) is published. The RCI gives a single figure (effectively a ranking) for each NHS provider organisation enabling comparisons of their activity with similar providers (for example, district general hospitals) and with providers in their local health economy. In most cases activity is measured in HRGs. For example an organisation with costs equal to the national average for its casemix will score 100; if it scores 125 it shows that costs are 25% above the national average and a score of 75 shows that its costs are 25% below the national average. For 2011/12, the RCI ranged from 74 to 167 although if mental health, community and single specialty trusts are set aside, the range was less marked – from 87 for Blackpool Teaching Hospitals NHS Foundation Trust to 118 for Mid Staffordshire NHS Foundation Trust.

A market forces factor (MFF) is also published to recognise the differences in costs in different geographical areas that are outside NHS control. Index scores are published pre and post application of the MFF. The post MFF index is the one generally used.

PbR tariff

Although reference costs are used to set the PbR tariff, there is a three year time delay to enable the tariff to be checked before being put into operation. As a result, costs submitted to the Department in July 2012 for the financial year 2011/12 will form the basis of the national tariff for 2014/15.

A number of technical adjustments are needed before national average costs can be turned into tariff prices. This includes traditional inflationary prices (pay and non-pay) as well as the costs of using new drugs, technology and techniques (for example, the cost of recommendations made by the National Institute for Health and Care Excellence – NICE). The inflationary uplift is then offset by an efficiency requirement. This means that providers are set a level of efficiency which must be achieved if they are to meet their financial targets at the latest tariff prices. See chapter 18 for more about PbR.

Patient Level Information and Costing Systems (PLICS)

Over recent years, systems have been developed at a more detailed level to identify and record the costs associated with treating individual patients. This provides organisations with an extremely rich source of data on which to base their activity and business plans. Patient level costing involves attributing the costs 'consumed' by an individual patient on a basis that is meaningful in clinical terms – in other words it is an approach that recognises that it is the clinical activity that leads to (or 'drives') the associated costs.

Benefits of PLICS

- An ability for an organisation to truly understand their economic and financial drivers and benchmark their services with other providers for productivity and efficiency
- A dramatic improvement in the clinical ownership of operating information
- The provision of crucial information to inform any future change in the grouping and classification of patients
- The provision of data to inform funding policy for payment of high and low outliers for each HRG
- The provision of valuable data in discussions with commissioners

PLICS represents a change in costing from a largely top down allocation approach, based on averages and apportionments, to a more direct system based on the costs associated with what actually happens to individual patients. Once costs have been identified at individual patient level, they can still be aggregated to HRG-level for wider comparison and to inform the national tariff. However, the intention is that over time the cost of treating each patient rather than average costs will be the main source of data for pricing models. A first step towards this long term aim was taken in 2013 when Monitor piloted (on a voluntary basis) a patient level cost collection for admitted patient care for acute providers based on the HFMA's costing standards.

More information about PLICS is available on both the Department of Health and HFMA websites.

Key Learning Points

- Costing involves quantifying the value of resources used to carry out an activity
- Costing is not an end in itself – it is used to help deliver improvements in healthcare services
- Costing information has many uses at both organisational and national level
- Monitor's *Approved Costing Guidance* sets out the principles and standards that NHS organisations should follow. It also contains guidance on reference cost collection and patient-level information and costing systems
- All costs in the NHS must be attributed to activities in a structured and logical way
- Costs are classified as direct, indirect or an overhead – here the focus is on how costs relate to what is being costed (the 'cost object')
- Costs can also be viewed in relation to how they behave – i.e. as fixed, semi-fixed or variable
- Clinical costing standards support a 'bottom-up' approach to costing and set out best practice for producing patient level costs
- Reference costs are collected each year and record activity levels, unit cost data and average length of stay for a range of specified activities. They provide useful management information and are used to develop the PbR tariff
- The currency used for the reference cost collection and PbR is the healthcare resource group (HRG)

- A national reference cost index is published each year – this allows comparisons between NHS organisations
- A market forces factor is published each year to recognise the impact of unavoidable cost differences across the country
- The intention is that over time information on the cost of treating patients will be used for pricing (rather than average costs).

References and Further Reading

Information about Payment by Results 2013/14:
https://www.gov.uk/government/organisations/department-of-health/series/payment-by-results-2013–14

Code of Conduct for Payment by Results, 2013/14, Department of Health, 2013:
https://www.gov.uk/government/uploads/system/uploads/attachment_data/file/141389/Code-of-Conduct-for-Payment-by-Results-in-2013–14.pdf.pdf

Approved Costing Guidance, Monitor: www.monitor-nhsft.gov.uk/costingguidance

Acute Health and Mental Health Clinical Costing Standards and MAQS templates, HFMA, 2013: www.hfma.org.uk/costing/

Information about healthcare resource groups, Health and Social Care Information Centre: www.hscic.gov.uk/hrg

HFMA Briefings on HRG4: www.hfma.org.uk/TrainingAndDevelopment/InformationServices/

Monitor guidance on service line management:
www.monitor-nhsft.gov.uk/developing-health-care-providers/service-line-management

Monitor guidance on service line reporting: www.monitor-nhsft.gov.uk/home/our-publications/browse-category/developing-foundation-trusts/service-line-management/service-l-5

Programme budgeting information: www.networks.nhs.uk/nhs-networks/commissioning-zone/support/reports-and-analysis/2011–12-programme-budgeting-data-now-available

Chapter 18: How NHS Services are paid for

> ## Overview
>
> We saw in chapter 10 that commissioners are allocated funding to purchase healthcare for local populations. The providers of those healthcare services are paid in line with contracts (see chapter 16). On average, about a third of this contracted patient activity is paid for under Payment by Results (PbR), the payment mechanism which currently covers the majority of acute hospital services in England. This chapter looks at what PbR is and how it works in practice and also covers how patient activity that falls outside the PbR regime is paid for.

What is Payment by Results?

Payment by results (PbR) is a system of financial flows (i.e. a mechanism for moving funds around the health service) that reimburses healthcare providers in England for the costs of providing treatment. Under PbR, payments made to providers of care for NHS patients, be they from the NHS, private or independent sector, are linked to the activity and services actually provided. Payment is based on a national tariff that links a pre-set price to a defined measure of output or activity while recognising the type, mix and severity of the treatment provided. In other words, the tariff for a particular treatment or procedure is the price paid by the commissioner.

Why was PbR Introduced?

PbR was a key element in the NHS reform agenda set out in the Labour Government's 2000 *NHS Plan*. The Government at the time wanted to be sure that the large increases in resources that it planned over a five year period would be used to develop and deliver more and better services. To achieve this aim there needed to be a financial system that contained the right balance of reward, incentive and equity – hence the introduction of PbR.

As well as paying providers of services for the actual number of procedures they carry out at the pre-set tariff rate, PbR also rewards efficiency. For example, if the cost to a provider of delivering a particular service is higher than the tariff paid, the provider needs to make savings as it is making a loss for every patient treated. If the provider's costs are lower than the tariff paid it makes a surplus which can be retained and reinvested in services including new staff, patient facilities, new technology or buildings.

The Basis for the PbR System

PbR is based around the use of a prospective tariff that links a pre-set price to a defined measure of output or activity. The two key issues are therefore:

- how is the activity measure defined?
- how is the tariff set?

How is the activity measure defined?

To have a tariff system it is important to decide what is being paid for – what is the unit of healthcare or 'currency'? The currency used for admitted patient care (covering a spell of care from admission to discharge), procedures undertaken in outpatients and accident and emergency attendances is the healthcare resource group (HRG). The currency for outpatient attendances is the attendance itself, split between first and follow-up attendances, the broad medical area (defined by a treatment function code) and whether the attendance relates to a single professional or a multi-professional team.

HRGs group services that are clinically similar and require similar resources for treatment and care. The latest version – HRG 4 – is 'setting independent' (i.e. the HRG applies for a procedure regardless of where it takes place) and supports the provision of components of healthcare outside of hospitals through the use of 'unbundled tariffs' (i.e. the payment or tariff can be split between different providers).

The currency used for adult mental health and learning disability services is the 'care cluster' which describes the common needs and problems of a group of patients over a period of time. Each of the 21 clusters includes a number of different diagnostic codes and there is a 'mental health clustering tool' to enable groups of cases to be identified. Contracts for 2013/14 are based on a price per cluster period.

How the tariff is set

A national set of prices (referred to as the 'tariff for reimbursement') is published annually, and is currently based on the average reference costs for HRGs as reported by providers of NHS funded services. Chapter 17 explains what reference costs are but in this section we are looking at how they are used to build the tariff. There is effectively a four stage process.

> **Building the Tariff**
>
> Stage 1 – activity is coded. Clinical coders assign diagnosis or procedure codes to activity based on the patient notes or discharge summary.
>
> Stage 2 – HRGs are assigned. Activity is automatically assigned to an HRG (via software called the grouper) based on the diagnosis or procedure codes – as logged by the clinical coder.
>
> Stage 3 – 'reference costs' are submitted to the Department of Health now (2012/13) and Monitor (from 2013/14).
>
> Stage 4 – the prospective national tariff is calculated. At present, this involves working out the national average cost for each HRG/service within the scope of PbR. For example, reference costs submitted to the Department in July 2012 for the financial year 2011/12 will be used to inform the 2014/15 national tariff. Tariff prices are adjusted (or 'uplifted') to reflect inflation, generic cost pressures, changes in technology and practice (for example, the cost of recommendations made by the National Institute for Health and Care Excellence

– NICE) and assumptions on efficiency improvements. For 2013/14 the tariff has been reduced by 1.1% – this means that the required efficiency improvement is greater than the increase to reflect cost pressures and inflation. At present, the Department of Health may also make a number of 'normative' changes to individual tariffs to correct known problems or to provide an incentive to drive a specific behaviour.

There are a number of other adjustments that can be made to the tariff that affect the final payment made to providers:

- marginal rate emergency tariff (MRET). A marginal rate of 30% of the tariff price is paid for emergency admissions above a set threshold
- short stay emergency adjustment. For patients admitted as emergencies that stay in for less than two days, the tariff is adjusted depending on the average length of stay for the relevant HRG
- long stay payment. Tariff payments are only intended to cover costs up to a nationally set length of stay for a particular HRG. For patients whose length of stay exceeds these 'trim points', providers may receive additional payments
- specialised service top-up payment. These top-up payments recognise the additional costs of undertaking specialised activity. Top ups for children's services, neurosciences, orthopaedics and spinal surgery are restricted to pre-identified specialist providers.

Cost Differences

As the tariff is currently based on the average cost of each HRG, providers receive either more or less than they need to cover their costs. There can be a number of reasons why costs vary including casemix (for example, a hospital that undertakes more of the higher cost procedures within a particular HRG may not cover its costs from a tariff based on average costs), clinical practice, local initiatives and market forces.

The area that generates most debate is the impact of market forces on an organisation's costs –organisations in some parts of the country have higher costs purely because their location means that labour, land, buildings and even equipment cost more. These differences are unavoidable and to ensure equity, a compensating adjustment is made. This adjustment is called the market forces factor or MFF. The most obvious area affected is London and the South East where the MFF can add up to 30% to the amount paid per patient.

Practical Application

The Department of Health issues guidance on how PbR should work in practice via a *Code of Conduct* aimed at all providers and commissioners, including those from the private or independent sectors. This Code outlines '…the principles that should govern organisational behaviour under PbR and set(s) expectations as to how the system should operate'. It aims to:

- 'establish core principles, with some ground rules for organisational behaviour, and expectations as to how the system should operate
- minimise disputes, as well as guide the resolution of them'.

A new version of the Code is published for each financial year and the 2013/14 Code is available on the Department's website.

How PbR has developed

Original plan

PbR was a fundamental change to the way money moved around the NHS and the original intention was that by 2008 all commissioning would be covered. However, a wide range of activities (amounting to two thirds of patient activity) remain outside the scope of PbR – most notably community and ambulance services.

Three models

The basic PbR model has developed to suit the different types of service. Following a major consultation on the future development of PbR during 2007/08[1] three possible models were identified:

* national currency and price (i.e. for services fully covered by PbR)
* national currency, local price (i.e. some services are not covered by reference costs so a national tariff cannot be calculated)
* local currency and price (i.e. where no suitable national currency yet exists).

National currency, local price

For some services, the introduction of a national mandatory currency provides a common basis for agreeing contracts alongside local flexibility to fit with the financial situation of the individual health economy. This model of national currency, local price currently covers the following:

* adult and neonatal critical care
* ambulance services
* HIV outpatient services
* specialist rehabilitation
* health assessments for looked after children placed out of area
* renal transplants
* adult mental health services (see earlier in this chapter).

It is envisaged that the speed with which new currencies are developed – as a route to expanding the scope of PbR – will continue to increase in the coming years.

Local currency and price

To be able to contract for healthcare services currently outside the scope of PbR in terms of both currency and price, providers and commissioners negotiate both the unit of

---

[1] *Options for the Future of Payment by Results: 2008/09 to 2010/11,* Department of Health.

healthcare and the price to be paid. Any local price needs to take account of the costs incurred by the provider so that they can afford to deliver the agreed level and quality of care. Local prices must be agreed formally, reviewed annually and established in line with the *Code of Conduct for PbR* (i.e. following the same approach as for services within the scope of PbR).

Quality

Another key factor affecting the development of PbR has been the focus on service quality and the use of best practice tariffs to reward high quality care. Best practice tariffs were first introduced in 2010/11 and reflect the costs of delivering treatments in line with NICE guidance (for example by undertaking cholecystectomies as a day case procedure or admitting stroke patients directly to a dedicated stroke unit). The standard tariff (i.e. *not* best practice) is set lower than the normal tariff price. An addition to this is then applied to give the best practice tariff. This creates a financial incentive for providers to adopt best practice patient pathways and treatments as those providers failing to deliver best practice will attract a lower payment for the activity. This approach is designed to deliver national improvements in the quality of care delivered.

Best Practice Tariffs 2013/14

- Acute stroke care
- Adult renal dialysis
- Cataracts (non-mandatory)
- 16 day case procedures
- Diabetic ketoacidosis and hypoglycaemia
- Early inflammatory arthritis
- Endoscopy procedures
- Fragility hip fracture
- Interventional radiology
- Major trauma
- 3 outpatient procedures
- Paediatric diabetes
- Paediatric epilepsy
- Parkinson's disease
- Pleural effusion
- Primary total hip and knee replacements
- Same day emergency care
- Transient ischaemic attack

Using PbR to influence

Increasingly, the tariff is used to influence the behaviour of those commissioning and providing healthcare services and to support the overall strategic aims of the NHS. For example, to help reduce emergency admissions to hospitals two refinements have been introduced to the tariff – as shown below:

Using PbR to Influence Behaviour

Emergency activity

Since 2010/11, providers of accident and emergency services have been paid at full tariff for the number of patients attending emergency departments up to the value of the activity recorded for the baseline financial year of 2008/09 priced at the tariff for the current year. However, attendances over and above this baseline are paid at a marginal or per patient rate of only 30% of tariff. Therefore, health economies where the accident and emergency admissions consistently exceed the contracted level have an incentive to redesign services and manage patient demand for those services. The money that commissioners would have spent on paying for the activity at full tariff is reserved to fund changes in the way emergency services are provided with proposals developed between commissioners and providers and overseen by 'urgent care boards'.

Re-admissions to hospital

In a similar vein, providers do not receive any further payment for a patient admitted within 30 days of their discharge following a previous admission if these 'readmissions' are deemed to be avoidable. In other words, hospitals are penalised if the patient is readmitted within a 30 day period if the readmission is related to the original reason for care and could have been avoided. The application of this 'rule' is subject to a locally agreed and evidenced threshold. Any resulting savings made by commissioners must be disclosed and reinvested to support patients following discharge from hospital. This applies to activity where a national tariff exists even if the patient is readmitted to a different hospital than the one where their original treatment was received. A number of patient groups are excluded including maternity, cancer, renal dialysis and paediatric patients.

What the Future Holds for PbR

Following the reorganisation of the NHS from April 2013, the Department of Health is no longer responsible for setting the PbR tariff. Instead (from 2014/15) prices will be set by Monitor in conjunction with NHS England. The development of currencies for pricing and payment will also be a joint responsibility, although NHS England will have primary responsibility for determining currencies. Together, Monitor and NHS England will decide which services should be subject to national tariffs.

All licensed healthcare providers will be required to comply with PbR and provide information to Monitor to support its development.

Alongside the changes in roles and responsibilities, the possibility of using costs from a sample of providers to set the tariff is being considered. Similarly, the expansion of the use of normative pricing – setting a tariff price based on a judgement about what efficiencies can be achieved or to encourage the take-up or dropping of particular treatments/activities – is also under review. The focus on quality is also set to continue with the introduction of 'annual packages of care' tariffs for long term conditions (for example, for cystic fibrosis);

pathway tariffs (for example, for the maternity pathway) and tariffs to support integrated care.

Paying for non-PbR Patient Activity

Block payments

For services that fall outside of the scope of PbR and the agreement of a local price per unit of activity, block payments are still in use, most notably for community healthcare services where a unit of healthcare may not easily be determined. Under a block payment approach, commissioners effectively pay healthcare providers a fixed amount of money for access to a defined range and volume of service for the year ahead. The provider receives an amount of funding irrespective of the number of patients treated or the type of treatment provided. Many of the risks in the system are therefore carried by providers. Rising activity levels increase provider costs, without generating additional income. Meanwhile commissioners face no additional financial costs if increasing numbers of patients are referred to the service provider. However, commissioners are not reimbursed if fewer patients are treated than originally planned.

Block payments are generally based on historical patterns of care and reflect the local costs of providing that care. As agreements are set at local prices negotiated between providers and commissioners, a commissioner's real purchasing power is affected by the relative costs – or efficiency – of the providers with whom they place their main contracts. This affects new social enterprise organisations (SEOs) established following the Department of Health's Transforming Community Services initiative as most of their income still comes from block contracts (see chapter 7 for more about SEOs).

Cost and volume

Cost and volume payments may also be used – here a fixed sum is paid for access to a defined range and volume of services but if there is a variation from the intended level of activity, there is a variation in payment levels according to a 'variation', or 'threshold agreement clause'. This determines the marginal rate of payment for higher or lower than target performance. The threshold agreement represents a mechanism for sharing the risk of unforeseen events between commissioner and service provider. Where this approach is used, the variation agreement tends not to be enforced within a narrow range of target activity. This band of activity is called the threshold or tolerance.

Cost per case

Cost per case payments identify for each episode or unit of care a payment to the service provider. Cost per case is commonplace where waiting list activity is placed with private sector providers, and for individual, expensive, and bespoke care package agreements (for example, the placement of patients in medium secure mental health facilities). Cost per case suits procedures that are infrequent, unpredictable, or can have significant cost variations. They are also used for treatments under the patient choice regime, where patients may choose a provider that the commissioner does not have an established contract with.

Whatever the payment type, all contracts agreed by commissioners with providers for NHS clinical care (except for primary care[2]) must follow the NHS Standard Contract (see chapter 16).

Key Learning Points

- On average one third of contracted patient activity is paid for under PbR
- PbR is a mechanism for moving money around the NHS and reimburses providers for the cost of treatments
- PbR uses a pre-set tariff for defined activities
- The unit of healthcare or the 'currency' used for admitted patient care, procedures in outpatients and A & E attendances is the HRG
- For outpatient attendances, the currency is the attendance and broad medical area
- For mental health and learning disability services the currency is the care cluster
- The tariff is based on average reference costs submitted each year by providers but there is a three year time lag before they are used
- There is a market forces factor to allow for unavoidable cost differences
- As well as the basic PbR model (national currency and price), there are two other approaches (national currency, local price and local currency and price)
- Increasingly best practice tariffs are being introduced to reward high quality care
- The tariff can be used to influence behaviour – notably to reduce emergency admissions
- Services that are not covered by PbR are paid for via block/cost and volume or cost per case payments
- The standard NHS contract is used for the commissioning of all NHS clinical services (except primary care) regardless of whether they are covered by PbR.

References and Further Reading

Information about PbR, Health and Social Care Information Centre:
www.hscic.gov.uk/article/2047/Introduction-to-Payment-by-Results

Information about healthcare resource groups, Health and Social Care Information Centre:
www.hscic.gov.uk/hrg

HFMA Briefings on HRG4: www.hfma.org.uk/TrainingAndDevelopment/InformationServices/

Department of Health guidance on PbR, including technical guidance and a mental health clustering booklet:
https://www.gov.uk/government/organisations/department-of-health/series/payment-by-results-2013–14

---

[2] The standard contract is not used for primary care services provided by GPs, dentists, opticians and community pharmacists as these are governed by separate contracts and form part of NHS England's direct commissioning activities – see chapters 4 and 6 for more details.

Code of Conduct for Payment by Results, 2013/14, Department of Health, 2013:
https://www.gov.uk/government/uploads/system/uploads/attachment_data/file/141389/Code-of-Conduct-for-Payment-by-Results-in-2013–14.pdf.pdf

Options for the Future of PbR – 2008/09 to 2010/11 (consultation paper and response) – Department of Health archived web pages: http://webarchive.nationalarchives.gov.uk/+/www.dh.gov.uk/en/Consultations/Responsestoconsultations/DH_082424

NHS Standard Contract 2013/14, NHS England: www.england.nhs.uk/nhs-standard-contract/

Information on urgent care boards, NHS England: www.england.nhs.uk/2013/05/09/sup-plan/

Chapter 19: NHS Charitable Funds

Overview

This chapter looks at the management of funds held on trust and is based on the legislative framework as it applies to England and Wales. The key Act is the *Charities Act 2011* which brings together all relevant charities legislation from previous years including Acts passed in 1992, 1993 and 2006. However, there are minor provisions in the old Acts that have not been consolidated into the *Charities Act 2011*.

History and Background

In 2012/13, there were around 280 NHS charities with a combined annual income of over £300m a year and £2.1 billion of assets. Following the abolition of primary care trusts in April 2013, the number of charities dropped to around 150 – although total overall income levels and assets remain unchanged.

To a large degree, the accumulation of these funds is a consequence of the historical funding of early health services through charitable sources. When the NHS was created, most existing charitable assets were pooled into the Hospital Endowments Fund. The main exceptions to this were teaching and university hospitals, which retained control of their endowments through Boards of Governors and management committees respectively.

Over the years, the NHS has been reorganised many times and laws passed to allow the charitable funds to transfer to NHS organisations that can use them for their intended purpose. More recently, funds have been boosted through capital growth and income from investments, legacies, donations and fundraising appeals.

The Nature and Purpose of Charitable Funds

A charitable fund is created when funds are accepted by a trustee to be held and used for the benefit of a beneficiary. The arrangement is usually governed by an instrument that sets out the terms of the trust and the purpose to which funds are to be applied by the trustee. In order to be deemed charitable, funds held on trust must exist to provide public benefit, be exclusively charitable and be used to further the funds' objectives. There are thirteen acceptable charitable purposes set down in legislation.[1] The Act also provides for the continuing admission of other categories that are analogous to these principal categories. The categories are subject to the overriding requirement of demonstrable public benefit. Funds that do not fall under one or more of the thirteen charitable purposes are likely to be non-charitable but if there is a doubt advice should be sought from the Charity Commission.

---

[1] These purposes were set out originally in the *Charities Act 2006*, since consolidated into the 2011 Act.

The Thirteen Charitable Purposes

1. The prevention or relief of poverty
2. The advancement of education
3. The advancement of religion
4. The advancement of health or saving lives
5. The advancement of citizenship or community development
6. The advancement of the arts, culture, heritage or science
7. The advancement of amateur sport
8. The advancement of human rights, conflict resolution or reconciliation or the promotion of religious or racial harmony or equality or diversity
9. The advancement of environmental protection or improvement
10. The relief of those in need by reason of youth, age, ill-health, disability, financial hardship or other disadvantage
11. The advancement of animal welfare
12. The promotion of the efficiency of the armed forces of the Crown, or of the efficiency of the police, fire and rescue service or ambulance services
13. Other purposes beneficial to the community not falling under any of the other headings.

There are three main types of charitable funds recognised in law:

- unrestricted funds – which may be spent at the discretion of the trustees in line with the charity's objectives
- restricted funds – which can only be spent in accordance with written restrictions imposed when the funds were donated or granted to or raised for the charity
- endowment funds – where capital funds are made available to a charity and trustees are legally required to invest or retain them. Endowment funds can be 'permanent' (i.e. trustees have no automatic power to spend the capital, only the income generated through its investment unless they apply for and are given consent by the Charity Commission) or 'expendable' (here capital can be converted to income).

Funds may also be 'designated' or 'earmarked' which means that trustees can set aside unrestricted funds for a specific purpose or more typically for an area of the hospital's operations – for example, cardiology, urology or nursing staff benefits. Designating funds can be useful where it is planned to build up funds through periodic transfers from unrestricted funds over time for a significant project or where funds are needed to meet on-going costs (for example, staffing) to which formal commitments have been made. It may also be a useful way to recognise the apparent 'wishes' of donors (which do not create 'restrictions').

Major public appeals may also be treated as an unrestricted designated fund – for example, an appeal to raise money for a cancer treatment building. Such an unrestricted fund will be a subsidiary registered charity (a special trust under Part 14 of the *Charities Act 2011*) under the umbrella registration of the NHS charity. The reason this can be treated as unrestricted is that the monies raised may be used on any of the costs of the project including building costs, professional fees, future maintenance costs (when specified in the subsidiary charity's objects clause) and meeting fundraising and administrative costs.

If trustees want to accumulate funds over a longer period (i.e. not for a specific project), they must request a 'power of accumulation' from the Charity Commission (unless the governing document already allows them to do so).

Charitable Funds Income

As we mentioned earlier, the origins of NHS charitable funds date back to pre-NHS days when early health services were funded largely by charity or through endowments. Over the years, funds have been added to gradually and today there are five main sources of new money for charitable funds.

Charitable Funds Income – Sources

- Donations
- Fundraising
- Legacies
- Investment income and interest
- Grants

In some circumstances income can also be generated through:

- trading – but only if it is in pursuance of the fund's primary purpose (for example, at a training course for NHS staff there may be an ancillary trade in refreshments)
- charging for part or all of a service provided by the fund (but only if it is for public benefit – the charges must not restrict benefits to those who can afford to pay).

We will now look at each of the five income sources in turn but first it is important to note that trustees are not obliged to receive funds on trust and may refuse where the conditions imposed by the donor are too onerous or where they are unlikely to be able to use funds as directed. To avoid criticism and safeguard their own position, trustees are advised to seek advice from the Charity Commission before refusing a donation. Acceptance of all donations should be tested against the general principle that it does not, nor appear to, place an NHS body or the Department of Health/Welsh Government under an inappropriate obligation.

Donations

Donations can be solicited (for example, through posters, leaflets or other appeals) or unsolicited (for example, where, at the end of a hospital stay, a patient asks how they can donate to the ward or hospital charity).

Donations of both types can be unrestricted or restricted. For example, an unrestricted donation would arise when a patient or relative gives money 'for the hospital charity' or 'for the ward funds' without specifying how it should be used. Even if there is a particular use suggested, it will only be a 'restriction' if the terms are strictly limited – for example, 'it must be used' or 'must only be used' – and are formalised in writing. A donation made in response to a fundraising leaflet soliciting donations for a general fund would also be unrestricted.

It is desirable to minimise the proportion of donations received as 'restricted' funds because this limits spending flexibilities. One way to do this is to use a standard form of receipt that invites donors to record how they 'wish' their donation to be used 'without imposing any trust'. The wishes expressed can be reflected through the designation of donations, but donations on these terms will be 'unrestricted'. The Charity Commission's *NHS Charities Guidance* includes a model receipt form as an appendix. Such a receipting system can also assist with accountability and the receipt can incorporate an invitation to donate under Gift Aid arrangements.

Fundraising

Fundraising income results from events (anything from coffee mornings and sponsored swims through to high profile celebrity events) and targeted appeals. If the money is sought for an explicit purpose (for example, if tickets or a poster for a charity dinner state 'all proceeds from this event will be used to buy monitors for the special care baby unit') then it must be used for that and nothing else. The power of NHS trustees to raise funds is set out in section 222 of the *NHS Act 2006* and the Act does permit funds to be used more flexibly where there is an insufficient response (a failed appeal) or an excess of funds over and above the appeal target, provided certain safeguards are met.

Legacies

Legacies can be restricted or unrestricted depending on the terms on which the bequest is made. The 'wishes' or 'desires' of a donor are normally non-binding designations, however reference should be made to the terms of the gift to ensure that a binding restriction does not mean that the legacy is restricted funds.

If the legacy cannot be fulfilled (for example, if the function it was intended for no longer exists or has been transferred to another body) the NHS trustee(s) concerned should consider whether they received the legacy under section 91 of the *NHS Act 1977* (re-enacted as section 218 of the *NHS Act 2006*), which may provide a power to redirect the funds. Advice may be sought from the Charity Commission. If it appears that section 218 does not apply then an application must be made to the Charity Commission for a scheme that allows the legacy to be used in another way.

Where a service transfers to another NHS body, the Department of Health or Welsh Government should be contacted, where appropriate, to organise a transfer of the related charitable funds. This is a separate issue from seeking the Charity Commission's authority to amend the trusts affecting restricted funds. Normally the service transfer (and consequent transfer of charitable funds) authorised by the Department of Health/Welsh Government would precede and inform the Charity Commission's decisions on how to amend the trusts of linked restricted funds.

The HFMA has issued guidance on how to account for the transfer of funds which is available on its website.

Investment income and interest

Where charitable funds have surplus monies not needed to fund immediate charitable activities, trustees may invest to generate additional income. However, they must do so in line with legislation and Charity Commission guidance. The relevant legislation is the *Trustee Act 2000* which includes a general power of investment that can be used in relation to any charity property held on trust (except property of charitable companies) subject to any 'restriction or exclusion' affecting the charity. This power allows a trustee to place funds in any kind of investment, excluding land, as though he or she was the absolute owner of those funds. The *Trustee Act 2000* also gives all charity trustees power to acquire freehold or leasehold land in the UK.

Investment income and interest (and any gains or investment losses) must be apportioned to the restricted fund that generates it. Where the trustee(s) administer(s) more than one charity, the income and investment gains and losses must also be apportioned to the respective charities. In the case of designated unrestricted funds of a charity the trustee(s) is permitted to apply investment gains for any of the objects of the charity concerned.

Grants

Grants are usually restricted income given for a specific purpose. As well as the general principles that apply to the use of (and accounting for) restricted funds, grants often have additional requirements attached. For example, how an acknowledgement is made in the accounts or other public documents.

Charitable Funds Spending

A charitable fund can only spend money in line with its charitable purpose. In other words, in the interests of the fund's beneficiaries (i.e. NHS patients) and not the NHS organisation to which it is linked.

Types of Trustee

The charitable fund's governing documents set out who or what controls, manages and administers the charity – these are the trustees. There are three main types of trustee in the NHS – corporate, special and appointed.

NHS Trustees – the three main types

Corporate trustees: most charitable funds in the NHS are managed by corporate trustees – in other words it is the NHS corporate body (i.e. an NHS trust or special health authority) that is the corporate trustee. The Board of the trust or authority acts on behalf of the corporate trustee in the administration of the charitable funds – the members of the Board are not themselves individual trustees.

Special trustees: under section 7 of the *1946 NHS Act* the endowment and trust funds were vested in the Board of Governors of designated teaching hospitals who acted as trustees. Subsequently the *1973 NHS Reorganisation Act* provided for the reorganisation of charitable funds held historically. Special trustees are no longer created.

Appointed bodies of individual trustees – under a number of different Acts, the Secretary of State for Health can appoint trustees to hold and administer the charitable funds associated with an NHS trust (often referred to as section 11 trustees); an NHS foundation trust (section 51 trustees); special health authorities; NHS England and clinical commissioning groups. In practice, these appointments are carried out by the NHS Trust Development Authority.

There are also two NHS charities that are governed by a charitable company limited by guarantee – here government ministers have the right to appoint non-executive directors.

It is important to appreciate that health service bodies are not themselves charities. Only the property they hold on trust for exclusively charitable purposes constitutes a charity. The decision as to which model of trusteeship should apply in any locality (and which NHS body, or body of NHS trustees should hold funds linked to a particular NHS trust or facility) lies with the Department of Health, exercising statutory responsibility (or Welsh ministers in Wales). The Department of Health operates a policy under which charitable funds linked to an NHS body are only allocated to its trusteeship if they total more than £500,000. Below that figure the trusteeship is usually allocated to another NHS body or body of NHS trustees that already holds more than £500,000 of charitable funds.

Trustees – Roles and Responsibilities

In broad terms, trustees have a duty to ensure compliance, a duty of prudence and a duty of care, each of which is discussed below.

Compliance

Trustees must ensure that:

- the charity complies with charity law and with the requirements of the Charity Commission as regulator. As part of this, they must ensure that the charity prepares its annual report, returns and accounts as required by law
- the charity does not breach any of the requirements or rules in its governing document
- any fundraising activity undertaken by or on behalf of the charity is properly undertaken and that funds are properly accounted for
- the charity's objects remain relevant and workable.

Duty of prudence

Trustees must:

- ensure the charity is and will remain solvent

- ensure the charity's income and property is applied solely for the purposes set out in its governing document and for no other purpose
- use charitable funds and assets wisely and only in furtherance of the charity's objects
- avoid activities that might place the charity, its assets or reputation at risk
- take special care when investing the charity's funds
- ensure adequate financial management and control arrangements are in place
- ensure the charity's expenditure is applied fairly amongst those who are qualified to benefit from it
- not allow the charity's income to accumulate unless there is a specific power of accumulation and a future use for it in mind
- have an agreed reserves policy that is reviewed regularly – unless this is done, trustees cannot be content that their reserves are at a level to meet current needs. If reserves are too high, the charity is retaining funds without justification and this could constitute a breach of trust. If reserves are too low, the fund's ability to meet future commitments or needs may be at risk.

Duty of care

Trustees must:

- exercise such care and skill as is reasonable in the circumstances having particular regard to any special knowledge or experience that he or she has (or professes to have) or that it is reasonable to expect of a person acting in the course of that kind of business or profession
- act with integrity and avoid any personal or organisational conflicts of interest
- ensure they have appropriate risk management plans in place. Trustees of charities with gross annual income over £500,000 must make a statement about this in their annual report
- consider using external professional advice where there may be a material risk to the charity.

The Charity Commission's guides *The Essential Trustee – an introduction* and *The Essential Trustee – what you need to know* are useful reference sources for all trustees (see the Commission's website).

Regulation – Roles and Responsibilities

At present, charitable funds are covered by both NHS and charities legislation. This 'dual regulation' can cause confusion and is currently (Spring 2013) under review by the Department of Health.[2] Until this process is concluded, key requirements for governance and finance will continue to be set by the Department of Health/Welsh Government and the Charity Commission. Their respective roles are set out below:

Department of Health

The Secretary of State for Health is responsible for bringing forward legislation on:

- the appointment and removal of trustees

---

[2] *Review of the Regulation and Governance of NHS Charities*, Department of Health, October 2012.

- the terms of their office
- the transfer of property between trustee bodies – as mentioned above, no transfers of charitable funds or trustee responsibilities can be made where NHS bodies are restructured without the Department's authority or agreement
- the preparation and audit of accounts for charitable funds – i.e. the overarching requirement to prepare accounts in line with the relevant charities acts and the SORP (see later in this chapter for details).

Welsh Government

In Wales Welsh ministers have equivalent powers to those of the Secretary of State in England, and exercise those responsibilities through the Welsh Government. The various provisions of the *NHS Act 2006* mentioned have parallel provisions for Wales, set out in the *NHS (Wales) Act 2006*.

Charity Commission

The Charity Commission is the statutory organisation that regulates charities in England and Wales. It is responsible for regulating the proper conduct and administration of charities. Its aim is to maintain public confidence in the integrity of charity which it does by encouraging better methods of administration, giving advice to trustees and investigating and correcting abuse. The Commission has the power to change the objectives of a charity where this is necessary and where trustees do not have the power to do so themselves. It also keeps a register of charities, which is open to public inspection.

The NHS is required to register charitable funds with the Charity Commission and to file audited accounts in a prescribed form and also to produce an annual report and annual return. The Charity Commission provides advice and guidance to help charities make effective use of their resources and to help trustees fulfil their objectives and obligations.

Charity Tribunal

The 2006 Act established the Charity Tribunal as an independent body to:

- hear appeals against decisions of the Charity Commission
- hear applications for review of decisions of the Charity Commission
- consider referrals from the Attorney General or the Charity Commission on points of law.

The Management of Charitable Funds

Day-to-day management

Trustees can only delegate authority that is specified in their governing instrument or section 11 of the *Trustee Act 2000*. However, they cannot delegate their statutory duties and responsibilities. This means that although in practice the day-to-day management of charitable funds may be delegated to a sub-committee and staff, trustees remain accountable for all decisions relating to the charity and its performance. It follows that they need to be well informed about the business of the charity if they are to meet their responsibilities effectively. They must therefore establish clear reporting lines and ensure that appropriate arrangements exist to enable them to oversee actions taken on their behalf.

This means that written rules and procedures must be in place covering the formal conduct of the charity's business. These will normally be set out in the form of standing orders, standing financial instructions and procedures or guidance notes, in addition to a 'scheme of delegation'. The frequency of trustee or committee meetings will depend on the size of the charitable funds being administered and the number and complexity of its transactions. Meetings need to be frequent enough to avoid any delays to the charity's administration that might lead to a failure to meet legal and regulatory requirements or to poor management of its resources.

When acting on behalf of corporate trustees, Boards of NHS bodies must recognise that:

- the charitable funds they are managing are distinct from the exchequer monies of the NHS body
- in acting on behalf of the corporate trustee they have separate and distinct responsibilities for the administration of the charitable funds.

This is best achieved either by:

- Boards meeting separately to deal with charitable funds business OR
- creating a separate committee to deal with matters relating to the charitable funds, and which reports to the full Board of the NHS body acting as corporate trustee.

The Charity Commission also encourages all charities to follow the advice set out in *Good Governance: a Code for the Voluntary and Community Sector* which identifies six key principles that trustees should adhere to in order to provide good governance and leadership.

Good Governance Code – Key Principles

- Understanding their role
- Ensuring delivery of organisational purpose
- Working effectively both as individuals and a team
- Exercising effective control
- Behaving with integrity
- Being open and accountable

Financial management

Trustees have a duty to use the income of their funds for the purpose for which they were given, unless the charity's governing document gives them the power to accumulate income or they have a specific application in mind. In order to justify the retention of income, trustees need to adopt expenditure plans. Budgets should be set with decision ceilings for fund managers and financial planning should be undertaken.

To be able to discharge their responsibilities effectively, trustees will need relevant management information to inform their decision-making. As well as the more usual financial information relating to budget and spend to date, trustees will need:

- to be informed of significant donations
- a list of large or significant transactions
- a summary investment report
- a report on slow moving or overdrawn funds
- a report on the use of the Chairperson's discretionary powers.

The Charity Commission booklet (CC60), *The Hallmarks of an Effective Charity*, sets out the standards the Commission believes an effective charity and its trustees will try to uphold and the principles that its regulatory framework exists to support. As such, it provides some useful pointers to trustees when reviewing their governance arrangements.

Risk management

Trustees should maintain a risk register and review it on a regular basis to ensure the effectiveness of actions taken to mitigate identified risks. Detailed guidance is available on the Charity Commission's website.

VAT

Value added tax in the NHS is treated quite differently from VAT in the commercial world. Essentially NHS bodies provide NHS services which are outside the scope of VAT (the VAT Act 1994) and thus their supplies are 'non-business'. However, many NHS bodies also carry out some limited taxable business activities (for example, non-contracted out car parking, catering, a reception shop). In the NHS body this gives rise to a partial exemption calculation which will include private patient activity (an exempt business activity). Furthermore, NHS bodies can recover input tax suffered for certain categories of contracted-out services (COS) just like central government public sector bodies.

All NHS bodies are technically registered into a group VAT registration (often called the NHS divisional registration) and when the charity connected to the NHS body has a corporate trustee (the NHS body) the charity, though a separate legal entity, becomes part of the group registration. Thus the COS rules also apply to the charity, as the charity is seen to be part of the NHS divisional registration.

In addition, there are special rules to zero-rate certain types of healthcare expenditure when the charity (not the NHS body) buys clinical equipment used in the diagnosis or treatment of patients or training of clinical staff or for medical research.[3] The entire cost must be met from

---

[3] VAT Act 1994 Schedule 8 Group 15 Charities.

charitable funds and the beneficiary must be a qualifying body. The supplier must sign a certificate from the NHS charity to confirm the arrangements. See also VAT Notice 701/ 6 March 1997, appendix F.

There are special VAT rules for charities when fundraising events are held depending on the frequency of such events and how the ticket price is determined, including the added complication of sponsorship deals. For more information contact HM Revenue and Customs.

Accounting Requirements

The detailed requirements for the preparation, audit and submission of annual accounts of individual charities that are not charitable companies depend upon their level of income and where they are based in the UK. The key document to refer to in England and Wales is *CC15 – Charity Reporting and Accounting: the Essentials*. This is available on the Charity Commission's website.

All charities with a gross annual income of over £250,000 in the financial year (and all charitable companies) must prepare their accounts on an accruals basis (i.e. all income and expenditure relating to the financial year is included in the accounts regardless of whether cash has actually been received or paid) **and** follow the *Statement of Recommended Practice (SORP) 2005* (also on the Commission's website). Below this threshold, charities may elect to prepare their accounts on a receipts and payments or accruals basis.

Trustees are also required to ensure that the charity keeps proper books and records.

As a minimum, all charities must:

- prepare and maintain accounting records which must be retained for at least 6 years
- prepare annual accounts and make these available to the public on request
- prepare a trustees' annual report and make it available to the public on request.

What Charity Accruals Accounts Comprise

- A statement of financial activities (SOFA) for the year that shows all incoming and outgoing resources and reconciles all changes in its funds
- A balance sheet, showing the recognised assets, liabilities and different categories of fund of the charity
- A cash flow statement if at least two of the following apply: the charity has an annual turnover of more than £6.5m; its balance sheet shows more than £3.26m gross assets; it employs an average of 50 or more staff
- Notes explaining the accounting policies adopted

Where charities have to account for more than one fund under their control, the accounts should provide a summary of the main funds. In particular, they should differentiate between unrestricted income funds, restricted income funds and endowment funds. The columnar format of the SOFA is designed to achieve this.

The Annual Report

The annual report is one of the key tools available to charities to help them communicate with stakeholders including donors, beneficiaries and the wider public. The SORP 2005 provides best practice recommendations, which in England, Wales and Scotland are underpinned by law. The annual report is normally presented along with the accounts but is legally a separate document. It should cover a range of information including, for example:

* details about how trustees are recruited and trained
* details about the charity's decision-making processes including, for example, what functions are delegated to sub-committees and staff
* an explanation of the charity's aims and the changes/difference it seeks to make through its work
* details of the charity's objectives for the year and strategy for meeting these
* details of significant activities, projects and services that contribute to the achievement of the charity's objectives
* details about reserves and grant making policies
* where material investments are held, details of the investment policy and objectives
* charities with gross annual income of at least £500,000 are required to report on their risk management plans
* plans for the future.

Guidance on the content of the annual report is available in Charity Commission booklet – CC15, *Charity Reporting and Accounting: the Essentials*.

Consolidation of Charitable Funds

From April 2013, a charitable fund's accounts will (under certain circumstances) be consolidated with the accounts of the NHS organisation to which it is linked. This is to comply with IAS 27 – *Consolidated and Separate Financial Statements*. This will not affect the requirement to submit accounts to the Charity Commission but it does mean that some charitable funds may also be asked to provide separate information to its linked NHS body. The Department of Health's review of the regulation and governance of NHS charities is likely to have an impact on the number of funds affected by consolidation as it is proposing that funds are transferred to new independent charities. If you want to know more about consolidation see the Charity Commission's website.

Key Learning Points

* There are around 150 NHS charities with combined assets of £2.1bn and annual income of over £300m
* To be charitable funds must exist to provide public benefit
* There are 13 acceptable charitable purposes
* There are three main types of charitable fund – restricted, unrestricted and endowment
* Charitable funds income comes from five main sources – donations; fundraising; legacies; investment income and interest and grants

- All charitable funds spending must be in line with its charitable purpose
- There are three main types of trustee in the NHS – corporate, special and appointed
- Trustees have a duty to ensure compliance, a duty of prudence and a duty of care
- At present, charitable funds are covered by both NHS and charities legislation but this is under review
- The Charity Commission is the statutory organisation that regulates all charities in England and Wales (not just NHS charitable funds)
- Trustees cannot delegate their statutory duties and responsibilities
- Charitable funds have written rules and procedures governing the formal conduct of their business including standing orders, standing financial instructions and schemes of delegation
- Charities with a gross annual income of more than £250,000 must prepare accruals accounts and follow the Charities SORP
- Charitable funds must produce an annual report which is normally presented with the annual accounts
- From April 2013, some charitable funds will be consolidated with those of their linked NHS organisations.

References and Further Reading

Charities Act 2011: www.legislation.gov.uk/ukpga/2011/25/contents/enacted

Other Acts of Parliament referred to in this chapter can be found via: www.opsi.gov.uk/acts.htm

The Charity Commission offers a range of useful free publications. These can be accessed via www.charity-commission.gov.uk or ordered from its offices. Guidance referred to in this chapter is listed below:

CC20 – Charities and Fundraising
CC3 and CC3A – The Essential Trustee: an Introduction and what you need to know
CC60 – The Hallmarks of an Effective Charity
CC15 – Charity Reporting and Accounting: the Essentials

Transfer of charitable funds guidance, HFMA, 2012:
www.charitycommission.gov.uk/Library/transfer_charitable_funds.pdf

Review of the Regulation and Governance of NHS Charities, Department of Health, October 2012:
https://www.gov.uk/government/uploads/system/uploads/attachment_data/file/127158/Executive-Summary2.pdf.pdf

The Charity Tribunal: www.justice.gov.uk/tribunals/charity

NHS Charitable Funds: A Practical Guide, HFMA, 2008: www.hfma.org.uk

Good Governance: a Code for the Voluntary and Community Sector:
www.charity-commission.gov.uk/Charity_requirements_guidance/Charity_governance/
Good_governance/governancecode.aspx

For VAT guidance, HM Revenue and Customs has a Public Bodies (NHS and Charities) Group,
contact details are:

Public Bodies Group,
Customer Coordinator Team,
Custom House,
The Dockland,
Pembroke Dock,
SA72 6TW.

There is also a charities email: charities@hmrc.gov.uk

Information about the Charities SORP 2005:
www.charitycommission.gov.uk/charity_requirements_guidance/Accounting_and_reporting/
Preparing_charity_accounts/sorp05docs.aspx

IAS 27 – Consolidated and Separate Financial statements, IASB: www.iasb.org/Home.htm

Chapter 20: Health and Social Care in Northern Ireland

Introduction

The primary difference between the NHS in England and services in Northern Ireland is that in Northern Ireland health services and social care are integrated. The Department of Health, Social Services and Public Safety (DHSSPS) is one of the 11 government departments formed to administer the responsibilities devolved to the Northern Ireland Assembly.

A lengthy review process that began in 2002 with the *Review of Public Administration* (RPA) resulted in the formation of a single commissioner, the Health and Social Care Board (HSCB), a multi-professional Public Health Agency (PHA), five local commissioning groups (LCGs) to cover the same geographical area as five health and social care trusts (HSC Trusts) and a smaller, more focussed Department. A regional Business Services Organisation (BSO) provides a range of business and administrative support functions for the health and social care service.

Who Does What?

The diagram that follows shows the structure of health and social care in Northern Ireland. The role of each key player is outlined below.

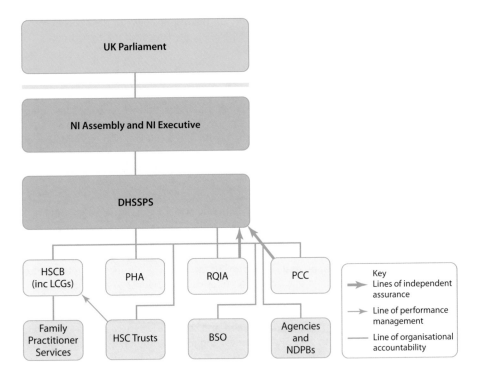

UK Parliament

The funds for running all public services in the UK ultimately come from Parliament and the public sector in Northern Ireland is expected to operate within the broad framework established by HM Treasury.

Northern Ireland Assembly

The Northern Ireland Assembly (NIA) is the devolved legislature of Northern Ireland. It has power to legislate in a wide range of areas that are not explicitly reserved to the Parliament of the United Kingdom, and to appoint the Northern Ireland Executive. The NIA consists of 108 democratically elected members.

Northern Ireland Executive

The Northern Ireland Executive is the executive arm of the NIA. It is answerable to the Assembly and consists of a Minster, Deputy First Minister and various ministers with individual portfolios and remits. Each minister is in charge of a Department and is responsible for its policy and business.

The Department of Health, Social Services and Public Safety (DHSSPS)

Health and social care (HSC) in Northern Ireland are the responsibility of the Minister for Health, Social Services and Public Safety. The DHSSPS is the largest of the departments established by the *Departments (NI) Order 1999*.

The DHSSPS's current remit covers policy and legislation relating to:

- health and social care (this includes hospitals, family practitioner services, community health and social services)
- public health (to promote and protect the health and wellbeing of the population of Northern Ireland)
- public safety (this includes the Fire and Rescue Service, food safety and emergency planning).

The Department's mission is to improve the health and social wellbeing of the people of Northern Ireland. It endeavours to do so by:

- leading a major programme of cross-government action to improve the health and wellbeing of the population and reduce health inequalities. This includes interventions involving health promotion and education to encourage people to adopt activities, behaviours and attitudes that lead to better health and wellbeing. The aim is a population which is much more engaged in ensuring its own health and wellbeing
- ensuring the provision of appropriate health and social care services, both in clinical settings such as hospitals and GPs' surgeries, and in the community through nursing, social work and other professional services.

The Permanent Secretary of the Department is also Chief Executive of the health and social care system, as well as Principal Accounting Officer for all the Department's responsibilities. Within the Department, the key business groups are the Resources and Performance Management Group; the Healthcare Policy Group; the Social Services Policy Group; the Health Estates Investment Group (HEIG); the Office of the Chief Medical Officer and the Office of Social Services. The Department also has a Modernisation Directorate and a Human Resources Directorate.

There are six professional groups within the Department, each led by a Chief Professional Officer:

- Chief Medical Officer Group
- Office of Social Services
- Nursing, Midwifery and Allied Health Professionals (AHP) Directorate
- Dental Services
- Pharmaceutical Advice and Services
- Health Estates.

Health and Social Care Board

The Health and Social Care Board (HSCB) (together with local commissioning groups – see below) is accountable to the Minister for translating his vision for health and social care into a range of services that deliver modern and effective outcomes for users, good value for the taxpayer and compliance with statutory obligations.

One of the key tasks for the HSCB is to ensure effective commissioning. The HSCB is also responsible for:

- performance management and service improvement – the process of monitoring health and social care performance against agreed objectives and targets and effectively addressing poor performance
- resource management – ensuring the best possible use of the resources of the health and social care system.

A full description of the responsibilities of the HSCB can be accessed from their website at www.hscboard.hscni.net/

Local commissioning groups (LCGs)

There are five LCGs:

- Belfast
- Northern
- South Eastern
- Southern
- Western.

Each LCG is a committee of the HSCB and is co-terminus with its respective Health and Social Care Trust area (see below).

LCGs are responsible for the commissioning of health and social care to address the care needs of their local population. They also have responsibility for assessing health and social care needs; planning health and social care to meet current and emerging needs; and securing the delivery of health and social care to meet assessed needs.

Public Health Agency

The Public Health Agency (PHA) has four primary functions:

- **improvement in health and social wellbeing** – influencing wider service commissioning, securing and making best use of resources
- **health protection** – protecting the community from any dangers to health and wellbeing
- **service development and screening** – working with the HSCB to provide professional input around safety and quality standards in commissioning care
- **HSC research and development** – promoting research and development into initiatives designed to improve health and wellbeing of the population of Northern Ireland.

Regulation and Quality Improvement Authority

The Regulation and Quality Improvement Authority (RQIA) is an independent health and social care regulatory body whose functions include promoting quality through disseminating best practice; regulating a wide range of health and social care services through registration, monitoring and inspection; reviewing and reporting on clinical and social care governance in health and social care and keeping the DHSSPS informed about the provision, availability and quality of health and social care services.

Patient and Client Council

The Patient and Client Council (PCC) is a regional body supported by five local offices operating within the same geographical areas as the five regional HSC Trusts. The overarching objective of the PCC is to provide a powerful, independent voice for patients, clients, carers, and communities on health and social care issues.

HSC Trusts

As mentioned, there are five HSC Trusts in Northern Ireland, offering a range of acute and community services. The Belfast, Northern, Southern, South Eastern and Western HSC Trusts were formed from the merger of eighteen health and social services trusts. A sixth Trust, the Northern Ireland Ambulance Service, manages the ambulance service for Northern Ireland. More information is available from the individual Trust websites which are listed at the end of this chapter.

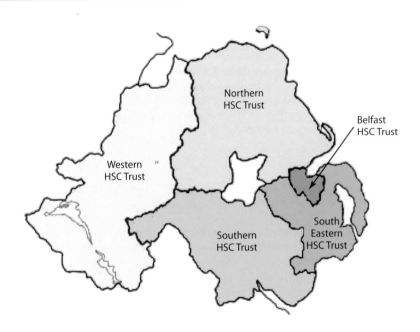

Business Services Organisation

The BSO provides a range of business and administrative support and specialist professional services to health and social care bodies – for example, financial services, human resources, information technology and procurement of goods and services.

Other HSC agencies and NDPBs

A variety of specialist functions are carried out by organisations on a Northern Ireland-wide basis. These include:

- Northern Ireland Blood Transfusion Service
- Northern Ireland Guardian Ad Litem Agency
- Northern Ireland Practice and Education Council
- Northern Ireland Medical and Dental Training Agency
- Northern Ireland Social Care Council.

Information on all the organisations referred to above can be accessed from the websites listed at the end of this chapter.

How HSC is Financed

As mentioned earlier, overall public sector funding for Northern Ireland is provided via the Northern Ireland block vote, as part of the national spending reviews. It is based on a population driven mathematical formula known as the Barnett Formula, which has been in use since 1979. Changes to the total provision for Northern Ireland are largely determined through

215

the principle of comparability, whereby the Treasury adjusts the Northern Ireland block vote in line with comparable programmes in England.

The NIA has the discretion to allocate devolved resources within the Northern Ireland block across all departmental spending programmes. The DHSSPS sets its proposed allocations in the context of the Minister's overall priorities and objectives for the Department's public expenditure programme. Spending on HSC equates to approximately 40% of the total public expenditure within the control of the NIA.

Revenue allocation

The DHSSPS makes direct revenue allocations to the HSCB and PHA to cover hospital, community health and social care services in the form of a revenue resource limit (RRL).

The HSCB and PHA use a weighted capitation revenue allocation formula to determine target allocations for hospital, community health and personal social services on a programme of care basis. The formula determines how much each of the five LCGs should receive to purchase services for its residents from HSC Trusts.

Substantial allocations are also given for the HSCB to commission the four family practitioner services (general medical, pharmacy, dental and ophthalmic services).

Budgets are set for each LCG area based on a weighted capitation formula. Performance against budget for each LCG area is closely monitored particularly in those areas of high expenditure such as prescribing.

As well as commissioning income, HSC Trusts may also receive income from:

- other government bodies or charitable organisations in the form of grants
- the DHSSPS to fund specific initiatives – for example, funding for professional training and development of nursing and social work staff
- charges to staff, visitors or patients – for example, catering, parking or private patient facilities
- recovering the costs incurred if a person treated after being involved in a road traffic accident subsequently makes a successful claim for personal injury compensation
- charitable donations for the sole benefit of and expenditure on patients. These charitable funds are accounted for totally separately from the funds which trusts are allocated for running their organisations and providing healthcare to their patients.

Capital allocation

The DHSSPS also receives a 'capital allocation' from the NIA – in 2012/13 this amounted to just under 6% of the total budget. Capital allocations are made directly to the HSCB, PHA, Trusts and smaller non-departmental bodies in the form of a capital resource limit (CRL).

Strategic capital planning is the responsibility of the DHSSPS. Individual HSC organisations submit business cases for capital requirements and these must be supported by the commissioner (HSCB) and submitted to DHSSPS for formal approval. Small elements of general capital funding are also made available to HSC organisations from the DHSSPS.

The DHSSPS is informed by, and contributes to, the overall 10 year *Investment Strategy for Northern Ireland* prepared by the Northern Ireland Executive. The current strategy covers the period 2008–2018.

How HSC Organisations Demonstrate Financial Accountability

HSC bodies have two statutory duties – to break even and to stay within their revenue and capital resource limits.

The HSCB and HSC Trusts prepare annual accounts in formats prescribed by the DHSSPS. Since 2009/10 they have been produced in line with guidance in the *Financial Reporting Manual* (FReM) which is based on international financial reporting standards (IFRS).

The DHSSPS issues a detailed *Manual of Accounts* for all health and social care bodies which is updated annually as required to reflect changes in reporting requirements. Where the guidance is not the same for each DHSSPS body, the manual sets out the procedures that each particular body has to follow.

The accounts must be formally adopted by the HSCB, in time to meet the NIA Summer recess deadlines (normally June following the financial year-end on March 31). Following this the accounts must be published on the websites of the HSC bodies, and made available to members of the public.

The Director of Finance is responsible for preparing the accounts.

The annual accounts are audited by the Northern Ireland Audit Office (NIAO), either by their own staff, or by contracting out to private sector firms of accountants and auditors. Each set of accounts is then formally laid before the NIA. The Assembly has a Public Accounts Committee (PAC) with a similar role to the committee of the House of Commons of the same name.

HSC bodies are required to have in place suitable internal audit arrangements. This service is provided on an in-service basis at present by BSO Internal Audit Unit. Internal audit must comply with HM Treasury's *Government Internal Audit Standards*. The adequacy of the internal audit arrangements is reviewed and reported on each year by the NIAO as part of their report to those charged with governance of each body.

How HSC Organisations are Regulated

As mentioned earlier, the key regulatory body in Northern Ireland is the Regulation and Quality Improvement Authority (RQIA).

How HSC Organisations are Structured and Run

The governance regime for HSC bodies is similar to that in place in the rest of the UK, including codes of conduct, accountability and openness, internal audit, external audit, board reports, annual accounts, annual reports and public board meetings.

As with the NHS in England, the Board of each HSC body is the pre-eminent governing body. There are also two mandatory committees of the Board – audit and remuneration.

Chief executives of HSC organisations are designated 'Accounting Officers'. They are accountable to the DHSSPS (and ultimately to NIA) for the appropriate stewardship of public money and assets and for the organisation's performance. Chief executives are also accountable to their Board for meeting its objectives and day-to-day running of the organisation.

Commissioning

As explained earlier, one of the key tasks of the HSCB is commissioning – the Board develops an annual commissioning plan in close partnership with the Public Health Agency and through a 'commissioning cycle' that covers:

- assessing needs
- strategic planning across HSC and all programmes of care
- priority setting
- securing resources to address needs
- agreeing with providers the delivery of appropriate services (and subsequent monitoring of that delivery)
- assuring that the safety and quality of services commissioned are improving, that recommendations from the RQIA and other reviews have been implemented and that as a minimum, services meet DHSSPS and other recognised standards
- evaluating impact and feeding back that assessment into the new baseline position in terms of how needs have changed.

For the most part the HSCB/ PHA commissioning plan reflects the decisions and recommendations of the LCGs as they have devolved responsibility for assessing and ultimately addressing the needs of their local populations, working within regional policy and strategy frameworks, available resources and performance targets. They also have responsibility for fully integrating commissioning to deliver better health and wellbeing and improve health outcomes for their local populations as well as reducing health inequalities locally and across the population of Northern Ireland.

As already highlighted these areas are co-terminus with HSC Trust boundaries.

A geographical orientation better reflects the needs of natural communities and the organisation of local health and social care economies, including hospitals, community networks and geographically based partners. On the other hand, commissioning around 'communities of interest' or client-groups, or 'programmes of care' can ensure that the needs of service users and carers are addressed holistically and services are planned in a coordinated way to meet particular needs.

Both approaches operate within the reformed health and social care commissioning landscape in Northern Ireland. Whilst the establishment of LCGs gives prominence to geography, this is balanced by 'programme of care' based planning within LCGs. These teams link across LCG boundaries where necessary, to form regional strategic planning networks relevant to client or 'community of interest' groups.

Commissioning of services from independent family practitioner contractors is managed by the HSCB. These arrangements recognise regional priorities, including service framework standards. LCGs identify local priorities and may use 'local enhanced services' as a mechanism for securing enhanced levels of service delivery.

Costing

The five locality based HSC Trusts submit annual 'reference cost returns' which capture the total cost of client and patient contacts spread across a prescribed list of health and social care activities.

Organisations can use these reference costs to compare their costs with those of similar organisations. This comparison establishes a benchmark which enables organisations to identify areas where they may be able to reduce costs or increase productivity by understanding and implementing best practice methodologies used in other provider organisations.

Charitable Funds

Charitable funds accounts are held by HSC Trusts in Northern Ireland and are derived, for example, from donations by individuals or legacies.

As in England and Wales these funds are used for the purpose for which the original donation was intended, or the bequest was made (where that is known) otherwise the uses to which the funds can be put may be unrestricted. Charitable funds are held and controlled by HSC Trusts and Boards as corporate trustees.

Northern Ireland's Charity Commission was established on 27 March 2009 and regulates charities, including HSC charitable funds. Details about the Charity Commission for Northern Ireland can be found at its website: www.charitycommissionni.org.uk

References and Further Reading

Department of Health Social Services and Public Safety: www.dhsspsni.gov.uk

The Health and Social Care Board: www.hscboard.hscni.net/

Public Health Agency: www.publichealth.hscni.net

Patient and Client Council: www.patientclientcouncil.hscni.net

Belfast Health and Social Care Trust: www.belfasttrust.hscni.net/

Northern Health and Social Care Trust: www.northerntrust.hscni.net/

Southern Health and Social Care Trust: www.southerntrust.hscni.net/

South Eastern Health and Social Care Trust: www.setrust.hscni.net/

Western Health and Social Care Trust: www.westerntrust.hscni.net/

Northern Ireland Ambulance Service Health and Social Care Trust: www.niamb.co.uk/

Northern Ireland Health Agencies: www.n-i.nhs.uk/index.php?link=agencies

Northern Ireland Medical and Dental Training Agency: www.nimdta.gov.uk/

Northern Ireland Social Care Council: www.niscc.info/

The Regulation and Quality Improvement Authority: www.rqia.org.uk/home/index.cfm

Health and Social Care in Northern Ireland: www.hscni.net/

Northern Ireland Audit Office: www.niauditoffice.gov.uk

Chapter 21: The NHS in Scotland

> ## Introduction
>
> In operational terms much of NHSScotland is similar to England and the underlying beliefs and fundamental principles of the NHS are the same. However, there are significant differences in the organisational structure, governance arrangements and approach to performance management, which are looked at in this chapter.

Key Differences

Key differences between Scotland and England are that:

- NHSScotland reports to the Scottish Parliament rather than the UK Parliament
- the Scottish Government Health and Social Care Directorate (SGHSCD) is part of the Scottish Government
- NHSScotland is part of the SGHSCD and consists of fourteen regional health boards, seven special health boards and one public health board
- regional health boards typically provide acute, mental health and community healthcare as well as managing primary care
- there is no regional tier in Scotland between the SGHSCD and the various health boards
- there are no NHS foundation trusts in Scotland as there is no provider/commissioner split.

Health Board Membership

Each health board is currently governed by a Board of Directors which includes non-executive members who are typically local authority councillors, representatives of Universities (where the health board is responsible for a teaching hospital) as well as lay members who are appointed for their expertise. Members of the Community Health Partnerships (CHPs) covering the health board's population are also represented on the Board. The composition of the Board will vary depending on the functions of the particular health board.

The Board of Directors also includes executive staff members – typically:

- a chief executive (who is also the Accountable Officer)
- a director of finance
- a medical director
- a nursing director
- a public health director.

This may change as the Scottish Parliament has passed *Health Board (Membership and Elections) (Scotland) Act 2009* which introduced elections for non-executive members of health boards on a pilot basis. The first elections took place on 10 June 2010 within NHS Dumfries and Galloway and NHS Fife. In NHS Grampian and NHS Lothian Health Boards there were two alternate pilot schemes which amended the approach to making appointments to health boards. At the time of writing, the pilots are being evaluated.

Development of NHSScotland's Current Structure

Partnership for Care – Scotland's Health White Paper (2003) was the blueprint for setting in place organisational and policy change within NHSScotland.

> **Partnership for Care – Key Features**
>
> * Dissolution of NHS trusts as separate legal entities and the transfer of their functions, staff and assets intact to new operating divisions of their local health boards
> * Introduction of a single local health plan
> * A new performance and accountability framework for NHSScotland
> * A revised financial framework and financial targets
> * Decentralisation of decision-making to front line staff

In 2005, the Scottish Executive Health Department issued *Delivering for Health*, as a response to the report from the group led by Professor David Kerr – *Building a Health Service Fit for the Future*. Both reports outlined future models of healthcare which move from acute based, episodic, reactive care to community-based, continuous, integrated and preventative care.

In 2007, the Scottish government launched *Better Health, Better Care* – this sets out a revised policy to continue the development of the NHS in Scotland. It is based on values of co-operation and collaboration and is aimed at tackling health inequalities, with patients at the centre of the NHS.

In 2010, the *Healthcare Quality Strategy for NHSScotland* set out 12 'quality outcome measures' to measure performance against the three objectives of providing a person centered, safe and effective NHS. These outcomes were aligned with the **H**ealth improvement, **E**fficiency and resources, **A**ccess, **T**reatment (HEAT) targets that each health board is required to meet.

In 2011, the *2020 Vision* was published which sets out the Scottish Parliament's vision for the future.

> **The 2020 Vision**
>
> * Integrated health and social care
> * A focus on prevention, anticipation and supported self-management
> * Where hospital treatment is required, and cannot be provided in a community setting, day case treatment will be the norm
> * Care will be provided to the highest standards of quality and safety, with the person at the centre of all decisions, whatever the setting
> * A focus on ensuring that people get back into their home or community environment as soon as appropriate

Statutory Provisions

The following legislation is relevant to the operation of NHSScotland:

* *National Health Service (Scotland) Act 1974* and *National Health Service (Scotland) Act 1978* – these Acts establish health boards and their roles and responsibilities

- *Public Finance and Accountability (Scotland) Act 2000* – this sets out the rules for the Parliament's budgetary process and procedures for the approval of expenditure, use of resources, management of audit and scrutiny of the outputs obtained from that expenditure
- *Community Care and Health (Scotland) Act 2002* – this provides the legislative backing for improvements in care services
- *National Health Service Reform (Scotland) Act 2004* – this allowed for the dissolution of NHS trusts and the establishment of CHPs; introduced a statutory duty for health boards to co-operate with each other with a view to enhancing the health of the nation (for example, through regional and national planning); established powers of intervention on behalf of Scottish ministers in case of service failure; and imposed on health boards duties to encourage public involvement and promote health improvement
- the *Patient Rights (Scotland) Act 2011* requires the Scottish Government to publish a charter of patient rights and responsibilities and keep it under review.

Who Does What – How NHSScotland is Structured

The First Minister for Scotland has responsibility for NHSScotland and is assisted by the Cabinet Secretary for Health and Wellbeing. The SGHSCD is responsible for NHSScotland and for the development and implementation of health and community care policy.

NHSScotland comprises fourteen regional health boards responsible for the protection and improvement of their population's health by commissioning and planning hospital and community health services. They are also responsible for the delivery of frontline healthcare services. The fourteen health boards cover the whole of Scotland. All health boards report to the Chief Executive of the SGHSCD.

In addition, there are seven special health boards and one public health board in Scotland which provide specialist and national services.

Health boards

In Scotland healthcare planning is primarily the function of health boards, although an overview is provided by the SGHSCD. Their roles and functions are summarised below:

Health Boards – Roles and Functions

Roles

- Improve and protect the health of local people
- Improve health services for local people
- Focus clearly on health outcomes and people's experience of their local NHS system
- Promote integrated health and community planning by working closely with other local organisations
- Provide a single focus of accountability for the performance of the local NHS system
- Involve the public in the design and delivery of healthcare services

Functions

- Strategic development
- Resource allocation
- Financial stewardship
- Implementation of the local health plan
- Performance management of the local NHS system
- Preparation and implementation of the local health plan
- Appointment, appraisal and remuneration of senior executives
- Governance of the local health board

Community health partnerships

All health boards are required to establish CHPs as committees or sub-committees. CHPs are largely co-terminus with local authority boundaries so there are, at the time of publication, 34 CHPs covering all 14 health boards and 32 local authorities. They are responsible for the development of community services in partnership with the local authority.

Local delivery plans

All health boards are required to publish a rolling three year local delivery plan (LDP). This means that it covers a three year period but is updated annually. The LDP is prepared by the health board in conjunction with the CHP, other local partners and local stakeholders. Each year, the SGHSCD issues guidance on national priorities and objectives.

What LDPs include

- HEAT targets and plans to meet them
- The health board's plans to contribute to national priorities
- Risk management plans
- Financial plans
- A summary of workforce requirements

Progress against the LDP is assessed throughout the year and a mid-year stock take of progress is undertaken by each health board with the SGHSCD.

Shared services

NHSScotland developed a shared service approach for payroll and financial services through a number of health board consortia. The shared service consortia supply these services to each of the NHSScotland organisations utilising a common chart of accounts and standard processes. This approach is now changing to a national system used by all health boards in Scotland and includes the 'National Single Instance Finance System'.

In 2011, a contract was signed for the provision of a single national human resources system for all health boards in Scotland. It is intended that the system will hold and manage employment information for all staff employed by all 22 health boards.

How the NHS in Scotland is Financed

NHSScotland funding forms part of the Scotland vote, which competes in the public expenditure survey (PES) against UK votes such as defence, social security and the environment. The First Minister for Scotland has the task of dividing up the Scottish vote among the various services for which he is responsible including health, prisons, education and social services. Health is one of the major areas of expenditure.

Since April 2009, the allocation of resources for hospital and community health services (HCHS) as well as GP prescribing is based on a funding formula developed by the NHSScotland Resource Allocation Committee (NRAC). This formula considers a number of factors including population share, the age and sex breakdown of that population and level of deprivation.

Since 2010, the work of NRAC has been undertaken by the Technical Advisory Group on Resource Allocation (TAGRA).

Cash limited/non-cash limited

Funds allocated for HCHS are distributed via a resource allocation. These are cash limited funds which mean that health boards are not allowed to overspend against their allocation (resource limit) and are highly restricted in their ability to carry forward surpluses or deficits from one year into another.

Funding for family health services (specifically, dental, pharmaceutical and ophthalmic services) forms part of the Scottish government health allocation. Although this is subject to a cash limit nationally much of the expenditure is not subject to cash limits at health board level.

Capital planning process

From 2011/12, the approach to managing NHSScotland's capital resources changed – as a result:

- less capital resources are distributed on a formula basis
- capital that is allocated by formula supports more routine spending and projects that fall within board delegated limits of between £1.5m and £5m
- all new projects above board delegated limits are subject to a bidding process for specific project funding.

Full details are set out in CEL 32(2010).

How Organisations Demonstrate Financial Accountability

Health boards are required by statute to operate within their:

- revenue resource limit
- capital resource limit
- cash requirement.

All health boards have a responsibility to control their finances throughout the year. Performance is monitored internally and externally by SGHSCD.

On an annual basis audited accounts must be produced and various statements signed by the Chief Executive, including an annual governance statement. The annual accounts must be published and made available publicly as part of the annual report.

Health boards are required to prepare their accounts in accordance with the *Scottish Public Finance Manual* which is consistent with HM Treasury's *Financial Reporting Manual*. The SGHSCD determines the format of external reporting by the production of an accounts template which is also used to produce consolidated accounts.

The principles of financial control and internal monitoring are set out in financial directions. It is left to local discretion to determine the exact nature of internal monitoring but it is sensible that this mirrors the external requirement. Internal financial control is ensured through the adoption of standing financial instructions, standard operating procedures and formal schemes of delegation.

Health boards meet regularly with the SGHSCD to monitor and forecast progress against the statutory targets. Where an organisation is forecast not to meet a target, remedial action is expected so that the target can be achieved. In cases where a health board fails to operate within the revenue resource limit set, then an adjustment is made in the following year's financial allocation to reflect the amount by which the board has overspent. The cumulative effect of successive years' failure to meet this target can be crippling for a board, as in the case of the NHS Argyll and Clyde Board, which the then Minister for Health took the decision to dissolve. The functions and services previously within Argyll and Clyde were subsumed within NHS Highland and NHS Greater Glasgow (now NHS Greater Glasgow and Clyde).

Governance and Audit

Audit Scotland and external audit

The audit of NHSScotland is the responsibility of the Auditor General for Scotland (AGS). The AGS appoints auditors to each health board. The AGS is supported by Audit Scotland, which commissions audits from its own staff and commercial firms of auditors.

Auditors perform the audits of health boards in accordance with the *Code of Audit Practice* issued by Audit Scotland and approved by the AGS. Auditors are responsible for considering:

- financial stewardship and governance through the annual audit of NHS bodies' accounts
- achievement of value for money through a programme of national performance audit reports.

Internal audit

Health boards maintain an internal audit function to carry out more detailed work at local level. Health boards may provide internal audit themselves, by means of a consortium arrangement with neighbouring boards, or contract out to private firms.

Counter fraud services

Counter Fraud Services (CFS) deters, detects and investigates frauds and other irregularities by family health service (FHS) contractors and patients against NHSScotland. CFS is hosted within the NHS National Services Scotland, and has links with every health board through partnership agreements and nominated fraud liaison officers. As partnership agreements develop, the role of CFS will extend to cover all aspects of boards' service delivery including acute hospitals and NHS staff.

Performance audits

Audit Scotland is responsible for carrying out performance audits (formerly known as value for money audits). The AGS also produces an annual overview of the performance of the NHS in Scotland, which provides information on a range of performance measures – clinical outcomes, waiting times, GP prescribing, health inequalities and financial performance.

Risk assessment

The clinical negligence and other risks indemnity scheme (CNORIS) was launched in 2000 with mandatory membership for all health bodies. The scheme has two principal aims:

- financial efficiency through cost effective risk pooling and claims management
- effective risk management by encouraging a rigorous approach to the treatment of risk.

Costing and Pricing

Costing

The *Costs Book* provides cost information for NHSScotland and a detailed analysis of where resources are spent. It is used mainly for benchmarking by healthcare providers to assess efficiency.

The *Costs Book* contains health board information for hospital and primary care services. There are three main reports:

- hospital sector – running costs
- community health services
- family health services.

Managers at all levels can use the information as an aid to decision-making, planning and control and it also provides a set of indicators of performance for comparison purposes.

The information contained within the reports is derived from financial and statistical information prepared by the health boards.

Tariffs

NHSScotland has introduced a tariff system for cross boundary activity flows for acute hospital in-patients and day cases.

The tariff is calculated using healthcare resource groups (HRGs) to reflect the differences in casemix complexity. The Scottish tariff relates directly to the *Costs Book* and is based on national average costs distributed over Scottish activity data. However, because the Scottish costing data is not collected at detailed HRG level, the English reference costs are used to estimate costs at the HRG level. This is done by applying relative weights to Scottish costs based on the assumption that the resource differential between any two procedures or conditions in Scotland is the same as in England. For example if a hip replacement costs around 4 times as much as an arthroscopy in England, then it is assumed that this is also the case in Scotland.

Although the Scottish tariffs are based on English HRG costs, they are not directly comparable due to the different methodologies applied.

Endowment Funds

As with trust or charitable funds in England and Wales, endowment funds are derived from donations by individuals, legacies etc. and are used for the purpose for which the original donation was given where that is known. Endowment funds are held and controlled by health board directors in their capacity as individual trustees. The board of trustees is an unincorporated body responsible for all matters relating to the charitable funds.

References and Further Reading

On line information from NHSScotland: www.show.scot.nhs.uk/

Health Board elections:
www.scotland.gov.uk/Topics/Health/NHS-Workforce/NHS-Boards/Elections

Our National Health: A Plan for Action, a Plan for Change, 2000:
www.scotland.gov.uk/Publications/2000/12/7770/File-1

Partnership for Care – Scotland's Health White Paper, 2003:
www.scotland.gov.uk/Publications/2003/02/16476/18730

Delivering for Health, 2005: www.scotland.gov.uk/Publications/2005/11/02102635/26356

Building a Health Service Fit for the Future, 2005:
www.scotland.gov.uk/Publications/2005/05/23141307/13104

Better Health, Better Care, 2008: www.scotland.gov.uk/Publications/2008/01/29152311/0

Healthcare Quality Strategy for NHSScotland, 2010:
www.scotland.gov.uk/Publications/2010/05/10102307/0

2020 Vision, 2011: www.scotland.gov.uk/Topics/Health/Policy/2020-Vision

NHS (Scotland) Act 1978: www.legislation.gov.uk/ukpga/1978/29/contents

Public Finance and Accountability (Scotland) Act 2000:
www.opsi.gov.uk/legislation/scotland/acts2000/asp_20000001_en_1

Community Care and Health (Scotland) Act 2002:
www.oqps.gov.uk/legislation/acts/acts2002/asp_20020005_en_1

National Health Service Reform (Scotland) Act 2004:
www.opsi.gov.uk/legislation/scotland/acts2004/asp_20040007_en_1

Patient Rights (Scotland) Act 2011: www.scotland.gov.uk/Topics/Health/Policy/Patients-Rights

Community Health Partnerships www.chp.scot.nhs.uk/

NHSScotland LDP guidance 2013/14:
www.scotland.gov.uk/Publications/2012/12/8405/downloads#res410447

Finance Shared Services, including the National Single Instance Finance System:
www.qihub.scot.nhs.uk/quality-and-efficiency/shared-services/finance-shared-services.aspx

Single national human resources system: www.swiss.scot.nhs.uk/index.php/eess

Technical Advisory Group on Resource Allocation (and NRAC reports):
www.tagra.scot.nhs.uk/index.html

Resource Allocation Formula for 2013/14: www.isdscotland.org/Health-Topics/Finance/
Publications/2012-12-18/2012-12-18-NRAC-Summary.pdf?45808047057

Arrangements for the management of NHSScotland Capital resources after 2010/11 – CEL 32
(2010): www.sehd.scot.nhs.uk/mels/CEL2010_32.pdf

Capital planning and investment: www.pcpd.scot.nhs.uk/Capital/CapIndex.html

Scottish Public Finance Manual: www.scotland.gov.uk/Topics/Government/Finance/spfm/Intro

Audit Scotland, AGS and the Accounts Commission: www.audit-scotland.gov.uk/about/ags/

NHS National Services Scotland: www.nhsnss.org

Counter Fraud Services: www.nhsnss.org/pages/services/counter_fraud_services.php

Clinical Negligence and Other Risks Indemnity Scheme (CNORIS): www.cnoris.com/

Scottish Health Service Costs Book, Information Services Division:
www.isdscotland.org/Health-Topics/Finance/Costs/

Scottish national tariff www.isdscotland.org/Health-Topics/Finance/Scottish-National-Tariff/

Chapter 22: The NHS in Wales

Introduction

The National Assembly for Wales and Welsh Government were established in 1999 and have devolved responsibility for a range of areas including health, education, agriculture, transport and local government. The Welsh Government develops and implements policy in these areas and is accountable to the National Assembly.

In terms of its structure, the Welsh Government comprises a cabinet of Welsh ministers led by the First Minister who is appointed by the Crown. Cabinet responsibility for the NHS in Wales rests with the Minister for Health and Social Services.

Following the referendum in March 2011, the Assembly has the power to create laws in 20 areas of devolved policy, including health.

Many of the principles underpinning NHS finance in Wales are similar to those in England – this chapter focuses on the key differences relating to finance and governance.

Health and Social Care Strategy in Wales

Together for Health

Together for Health is the five year vision for the NHS in Wales published in Autumn 2011. The Welsh Government's website makes clear that 'it is based around community services with patients at the centre, and places prevention, quality and transparency at the heart of healthcare'. The aim is for Wales to have health and healthcare services matching the best anywhere, and that by 2016:

- health will be better for everyone in Wales
- access and patient experience will be better
- better service safety and quality will improve health outcomes.

The main commitments in *Together for Health* are:

- service modernisation, including more care provided closer to home and specialist 'centres of excellence'
- addressing health inequalities
- better IT systems and an information strategy ensuring improved care for patients
- improving quality of care
- workforce development
- instigating a 'compact with the public'
- a changed financial regime.

Achieving Excellence – the Quality Delivery Plan for the NHS in Wales 2012 – 2016 sets out in detail how the aims in *Together for Health* will be achieved. Its focus is on quality improvement and quality assurance.

Programme for Government

Programme for Government is the Welsh Government's plan for the fourth Assembly until 2016. It is intended to focus on delivery and will measure success by the impact it has on people's lives. In relation to health services, the Programme has an overall aim of ensuring better health for all with reduced health inequalities under the theme of '21st Century Healthcare'. The key actions are:

- improving health outcomes by ensuring the quality and safety of services is enhanced
- improving access and patient experiences
- preventing poor health and reducing health inequalities.

Progress on delivering the aim of the *Programme for Government* is being measured through tracking a number of outcome indicators.

Who Does What?

The diagram that follows shows the structure of the NHS in Wales and how accountability flows. Each element is discussed in more detail below.

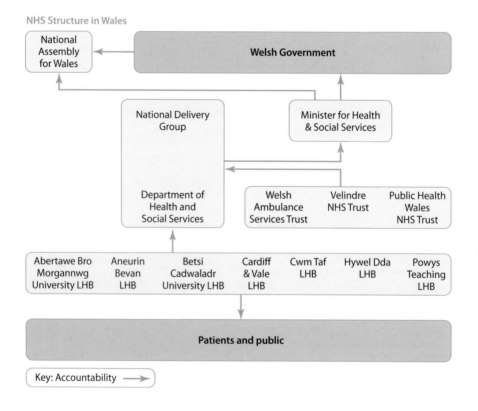

NHS Structure in Wales

National Assembly for Wales

The National Assembly for Wales is the democratically elected body that represents the interests of Wales and its people, makes laws for Wales, and holds the Welsh Government to account. It comprises 60 members, known as Assembly Members, or AMs.

The Welsh Government

The Welsh Government is responsible for setting overall policy for the NHS in Wales and for funding the local health boards (LHBs).

The arrangements provided for in the *Government of Wales Act 2006* created a formal legal separation between the National Assembly for Wales, the legislature comprising the 60 Assembly members, and the Welsh Government, the executive, comprising the First Minister, Welsh ministers, Deputy Welsh ministers and the Counsel General. The role of the executive is to:

- make decisions
- develop and implement policy
- exercise executive functions
- make statutory instruments.

The AMs scrutinise the Welsh Government's decisions and policies, hold ministers to account, approve budgets for the Welsh Government's programmes, and have the power to enact 'Assembly Measures' on certain matters.

Minister for Health and Social Services

The Minister for Health and Social Services is responsible for and accountable to the National Assembly for Wales for the exercise of all the powers in the health and social services portfolio.

National Delivery Group

The Chief Executive of NHS Wales is responsible for providing the Minister with policy advice and exercising strategic leadership and management of the NHS. To support this role, the Chief Executive (also known as the Director General) chairs a National Delivery Group, which forms part of the Department of Health and Social Services.

This group is responsible for overseeing the development and delivery of NHS services across Wales and for planning and performance management of the NHS on behalf of Welsh ministers. This is in accordance with the directions set by the Minister.

Department of Health and Social Services

The Department of Health and Social Services supports the Minister and the Director General in discharging their responsibilities. The Chief Medical Officer for Wales is also a member of the Department of Health and Social Services.

The role of the Department is to set and implement policy in relation to:

- planning, developing and co-ordinating the delivery of NHS services, including specialist services, within the framework set down by the Minister
- defining, in consultation with NHS local bodies, required outcomes and accompanying resources as part of a regular planning cycle
- facilitating the effective performance management of NHS local bodies to ensure delivery of defined outcomes.

The Department is also responsible for the development of social services policy for Wales.

The NHS in Wales

The NHS in Wales comprises seven local health boards (LHBs) and three NHS trusts. Specialist services are planned and funded jointly by the LHBs through the Welsh Health Specialised Services Committee.

The LHBs and trusts are accountable to the Director General of Health and Social Services through their chief executives. The Director General is in turn accountable to the Minister for Health and Social Services.

Local health boards

The seven LHBs are responsible for delivering all healthcare services within a geographical area. In particular they are responsible for:

- planning, designing, developing and securing delivery of primary, community and secondary care services
- specialist and tertiary services for their areas, to meet identified local needs within the national policy and standards framework set out by the Minister.

The LHBs adhere to the standards of good governance set for the NHS in Wales, which are based on the Assembly Government's *Citizen Centred Governance Principles*.

LHBs have a statutory financial duty to keep within their revenue and capital resource limits. In addition they are expected to achieve a 95% compliance rate with the *Better Payment Practice Code*.

NHS trusts

There are three NHS trusts in Wales:

- the Welsh Ambulance Services NHS Trust provides emergency and non-emergency ambulance services and manages NHS Direct in Wales
- Velindre NHS Trust provides specialist cancer services for South Wales, as well as hosting several all-Wales services, including the Welsh Blood Service and the NHS Wales Informatics Service

- Public Health Wales NHS Trust – provides all-Wales screening services and a National Public Health Service.

NHS trusts have a statutory duty to break even, which is measured on an annual basis. They are also expected to keep within their capital resource limits and external financing limits and achieve a 95% compliance rate with the *Better Payment Practice Code*.

How the NHS in Wales is Funded

NHS Wales is funded by the Welsh Government which itself receives funds voted to it by the UK Parliament.

Any changes to the funding provided to the Department of Health for the NHS in England are matched by an increase in the Welsh Government's funding through the Barnett formula, but it is for the Welsh Government to determine how this funding is applied. This is done through an annual budget planning round which allocates funding to the sectors for which the Welsh Government has responsibility. The budget is formally presented to the Assembly for approval in an annual budget motion.

NHS Wales receives its funding allocation from the Welsh Government's Health, Social Services and Children's budget which is the largest expenditure group and accounts for approximately 40% of the Assembly's total budget.

The allocation comprises:

- a revenue budget for current expenditure (i.e. the day-to-day money for salaries and consumables) – this amounted to £5.941bn in 2012/13
- a capital budget for expenditure on larger, long life items such as land and buildings – a total of £220m in 2012/13.

The Welsh Government holds back a 'top slice' for centrally funded initiatives or services (such as the costs of training new doctors and nurses). It then decides how to share the rest of the allocations to NHS organisations.

Revenue allocation

Each health board has a unified allocation to fund healthcare for its population. The allocation for hospital and community health services is based on resident populations. Allocations for general medical services and prescribing are based on registered populations, and pharmacy and dental contract allocations are based on provision of services.

The distribution of funding is largely based on historical patterns. A needs based allocation formula was developed by the late Professor Townsend in 2001 to allocate funding based on the health needs of the local population. The formula takes as its base the population covered by a health board area and then adjusts that total to take account of:

- the health needs of the population

- unavoidable geographical variations in the cost of services.

Implementation of the formula has been limited to date. A review of resource allocation is planned as part of the work on a finance regime – one of the commitments in *Together for Health*.

LHBs contribute to the Welsh Health Specialised Services Committee (WHSSC), which is responsible for planning and funding specialised services on behalf of the health boards.

The Welsh Ambulance Services NHS Trust and Velindre NHS Trust receive their funding through 'healthcare agreements' with the LHBs and some funding via WHSSC.

The Public Health Wales NHS Trust receives the majority of its funding directly from the Welsh Government.

At the time of writing (April 2013) a review of the Welsh Ambulance Services NHS Trust was underway which includes its funding arrangements.

As well as the Welsh Government revenue allocation, healthcare agreements with other LHBs and cross border income, LHBs may also receive funding from:

- the leasing of buildings
- charges to staff, visitors or patients (for example, catering or private patient facilities)
- the Welsh Government for specific initiatives, teaching and research and development
- grants from government bodies.

Capital allocation

In 2012/13 the capital budget was £220 million, which accounts for just under 4% of the total health budget. The Welsh Government allocates these 'capital' resources to LHBs and NHS trusts. There are 2 types:

- discretionary capital to cover routine equipment replacement; IT developments and small-scale building works
- all Wales Capital Programme Funding for specific medium to large scale schemes beyond the scope of discretionary capital.

LHBs and trusts are required to submit business cases for funding for major capital schemes using the *Five Case Model*. The Department of Health and Social Services has established an Investment Policy and Appraisal Group (IPAG) to provide support to LHBs and trusts in the development of business cases, and also to scrutinise cases at all stages of their development.

NHS trusts are allowed to retain sale proceeds from the disposal of assets up to a maximum of £500,000.

As with other parts of the public sector, the Welsh Government and NHS Wales are not able to vire funds between capital and revenue allocations.

The private finance initiative is no longer used in Wales although a small number of schemes still exist.

How the NHS in Wales Demonstrates Financial Accountability

The financial performance of NHS organisations in Wales is assessed using the following targets:

- break even performance for NHS trusts or resource limit for LHBs (the break even duty)
- external financing limit for NHS trusts (the difference between what a trust plans to spend on capital in a year and the level of funding that it has available internally)
- best practice cash balance for LHBs – the Welsh Government has a best practice closing cash balance guide equivalent to 1/300th of the total revenue and capital resource limits. It is good practice to achieve a closing cash balance of as close to zero as possible to demonstrate that the health board is not receiving cash ahead of need
- capital resource limits for LHBs and NHS trusts
- creditor payments (95% of non-NHS creditors, based on the number of bills, must be paid within 30 days of delivery or receipt of a valid invoice whichever is sooner).

The format and presentation of statutory accounts for the NHS in Wales is similar to that for trusts in England. The Welsh Government produces separate *Manuals for Accounts* for LHBs and NHS trusts. The accounts must be adopted formally by the Board and presented at the annual general meeting by 30 September following the financial year end on 31 March.

The Director of Finance is responsible for preparing the accounts.

The individual accounts of LHBs and NHS trusts are summarised into two consolidated NHS accounts that are then subject to independent audit and scrutiny by the Wales Audit Office.

Each NHS organisation is also required to submit monthly monitoring statements reporting on actual financial performance and forecast outturn. This is supplemented by a detailed commentary from the Director of Finance detailing assumptions and risks behind the reported position. The overall position is monitored by the Welsh Government. The Minister will occasionally make a statement to the Assembly on the financial position of the NHS in Wales.

How the NHS in Wales is Regulated

Performance management

Performance management of NHS Wales organisations is undertaken by the Department of Health and Social Services, and follows six key principles:

- self-governance
- proportionality
- transparency
- openness
- minimal duplication
- minimal information.

The Department is supported by a 'Delivery Unit' in relation to performance management and improvement of NHS Wales organisations.

Audit

The external audit arrangements in Wales are different to England. The Wales Audit Office was created in April 2005 and the Auditor General for Wales is now responsible for auditing all public accounts and laying them before the Assembly.

Each NHS organisation is responsible for providing an effective internal audit service to meet NHS minimum audit standards. All NHS bodies are required to submit a governance statement as part of their annual accounts. Accountable officers (i.e. chief executives) are required to sign the statement on behalf of the board.

Standards

In May 2005, the Welsh Government published the *Healthcare Standards for Wales*. These provided a common framework to support the NHS and partner organisations in providing effective, timely and quality services across all healthcare settings. The standards were used by the Healthcare Inspectorate Wales (HIW) as part of their processes for assessing the quality, safety and effectiveness of healthcare providers and commissioners across Wales. Existing Welsh risk management standards, which were developed by the Welsh Risk Pool, were incorporated into the self-assessment process for the *Healthcare Standards* during 2007. In April 2010, a revised set of standards was issued following a consultation process – the standards, *Doing Well, Doing Better: Standards for Health Services in Wales* replace the *Healthcare Standards for Wales* framework and came into effect from 1st April 2010.

How NHS Organisations in Wales are Structured and Run

For the NHS in Wales, governance is defined as 'A system of accountability to citizens, service users, stakeholders and the wider community, within which healthcare organisations work, take decisions and lead their people to achieve their objectives.'

As in England, all NHS organisations have a Board which is the pre-eminent governing body and which has some functions 'reserved' to it (including financial stewardship, strategy and appointing senior executives). However, Boards are also required to establish (as a minimum) a number of committees to cover the following aspects of business:

* quality and safety
* audit
* information governance
* charitable funds
* remuneration and terms of service
* Mental Health Act requirements.

As in England, NHS bodies must have an 'Accountable Officer' (the chief executive) who is accountable to the Welsh Government for the proper stewardship of public money and assets and for the organisation's performance. Chief executives are also accountable to their own Board for meeting its objectives and the day-to-day running of the organisation.

The *Codes of Conduct and Accountability* and the *Code of Conduct for NHS Managers* apply in Wales, although they are under review.

Commissioning

LHBs are responsible for deciding how to use their funding to meet the health needs of their population including hospital, community, GP and other primary care services. LHBs also fund services provided by the private and independent sectors although the Welsh Government is committed to eliminating the use of private sector hospitals.

LHBs also contribute to the WHSSC, which plans and funds specialised services on behalf of the boards. The WHSSC decides how to use its funding to meet the specialist health needs of the whole Welsh population.

Patient flows between LHBs are funded through healthcare agreements between the boards. These are currently based on historic costs, but consideration is being given to introducing an all-Wales standard price for activity.

Although LHBs have a large amount of discretion in relation to how they use their funding, they must meet the priorities set out in the *Delivery Framework* issued by the Welsh Government.

Costing

Since 2009/10, costs have been based on the version 4 HRG grouper and costing of provider services has been a requirement for LHBs. LHBs are also required to analyse costs over the 23 programme budget categories, based on version 10 of the *International Classification of Diseases*.

The Welsh Government has mandated the implementation of service line reporting (SLR) in NHS organisations in Wales.

The development of costing in NHS Wales is overseen by a Financial Information and Costing Group, which is a sub-group of the NHS Wales Directors of Finance Group.

How Services are paid for

As mentioned above, patient flows between LHBs are funded through healthcare agreements between the boards. These are currently based on historic costs, but consideration is being given to introducing an all-Wales standard cost for paying for activity. Healthcare agreements also cover funding allocated by the WHSSC to specialised services health board providers.

Treatment for some Welsh residents, particularly for specialised services and patients living in North Wales and Powys, is provided by English NHS providers. These treatments are funded through contracts with the English provider. Where applicable, payment is based on the Payment by Results English tariff (see chapter 18 for more about PbR).

Charitable Funds

Charitable funds are held by NHS trusts and health boards in Wales under the same legislative framework as exists in England. All funds are registered with the Charity Commission and accounts must be submitted to the Charity Commission.

See chapter 19 for more about charitable funds in England and Wales.

References and Further Reading

Welsh Government health and social care web pages:
http://new.wales.gov.uk/topics/health/?lang=en

Health in Wales Information Service: www.wales.nhs.uk

Together for Health, Welsh Government, 2012:
http://wales.gov.uk/topics/health/publications/health/reports/together/?lang=en

Achieving Excellence – the Quality Delivery Plan for the NHS in Wales 2012 – 2016, Welsh Government, 2013:
http://wales.gov.uk/topics/health/publications/health/strategies/excellence/?lang=en

Programme for Government, Welsh Government: http://wales.gov.uk/about/programmeforgov/;jsessionid=5DB6E3D2F8EAC567EA457B6127CF6837?lang=en

NHS Wales Governance e-Manual (including the NHS Wales Act 2006 and Citizen Centred Governance Principles): www.nhswalesgovernance.com/display/home.aspx

Codes of Conduct and Accountability (part of the Governance e-Manual):
www.nhswalesgovernance.com/display/Home.aspx?a=244&s=13&m=69&d=0&p=0

Better Payment Practice Code: www.payontime.co.uk/

The Five Case Model: www.hm-treasury.gov.uk/data_greenbook_business.htm

Wales Audit Office: www.wao.gov.uk/

Accounting guidance for LHBs and Trusts (part of the Governance e-Manual):
www.nhswalesgovernance.com/display/Home.aspx?a=536&s=39&m=296&d=0&p=338

Healthcare Inspectorate Wales: www.hiw.org.uk/

Doing Well, Doing Better: Standards for Health Services in Wales, 2010 (part of the governance e-Manual): www.nhswalesgovernance.com/display/Home.aspx?a=130&s=2&m=0&d=0&p=0

Programme budgeting (Wales): http://wales.gov.uk/topics/statistics/headlines/health2013/nhs-expenditure-programme-budgets-2011-12/?lang=en

Appendix 1: The 'Old' Primary Care Trust (PCT) Allocation Process

> Overview
>
> This appendix is designed to give you an idea of how a formula is used to allocate resources by summarising the approach used to distribute funding to PCTs up until 2012/13.

PCT Allocations

There were four elements that affected PCTs' allocations:

1. By far the most important was the **recurrent baseline** (a) – the prior year's allocation.

2. **Weighted capitation targets** (b) – targets were set according to the national 'weighted capitation formula' (see below), which calculated PCTs' 'fair shares' of available resources based on the health needs of their populations. These targets were re-calculated regularly prior to the allocation of resources to take account of changes such as the latest census data. Changes in the targets did not immediately lead to changes in actual allocations.

3. **Distance from target** (DFT) – this was the difference between (a) and (b); if (b) was greater than (a) a PCT was said to be under target; if (b) was less than (a) it was said to be over target. These were expressed in monetary and percentage terms.

4. **Pace of change** – this was the speed at which PCTs were moved closer to target (or 'levelled up'). This was achieved through the distribution of extra resources – a process known as differential growth, where all PCTs received some growth funds, but higher levels of growth were targeted at PCTs most under target. PCTs did not receive their target allocation immediately but were moved to it over a number of years.

The Weighted Capitation Formula

As healthcare is provided to people, the primary determinant of a PCT's funding allocation was the size of its population. However, because a simple capitation formula (i.e. an amount per head) would provide the same level of funding for every person in the population, adjustments were needed to reflect the fact that the healthcare requirements of an individual depended on a range of factors including their age and needs. The makeup of each PCT's population varied and so the population for a PCT was 'weighted' (or adjusted) for:

- age related need – recognising that levels of demand for health services vary according to the age structure of the population
- additional need – reflecting relative need for healthcare over and above that accounted for by age
- unavoidable costs – taking account of unavoidable geographical variations in the cost of providing services.

PCTs then received the same level of funding per weighted head of population.

Components of the formula

The weighted capitation formula considered relative need in separate areas with each component given a relative weighting to reflect the makeup of overall health spending. There were three components as set out below – the figures in brackets were the relative weights (they do not total 100% due to roundings):

- hospital and community health services (HCHS) (76%)
- prescribing – the drugs bill (12%)
- primary medical services (11%).

A similar approach was followed for each component – in effect a weighted population was calculated for each component and these individual weighted populations were combined in the set proportions (76%, 12% and 11%) to create a unified weighted population.

Appendix 2: Abbreviations

This list includes only abbreviations that have been used in this Guide. If you want to consult a more extensive list that records acronyms used in the NHS over the years, go to the publications and guidance pages of the HFMA's website:
www.hfma.org.uk/publications-and-guidance/

ABC	Activity Based Costing
ACRA	Advisory Committee on Resource Allocation
AGS	Auditor General Scotland
AHP	Allied Health Professionals
ALB	Arm's Length Body
AM	Assembly Member (Wales)
AME	Annually Managed Expenditure
APMS	Alternative Provider Medical Services
AQP	Any Qualified Provider
ASB	Accounting Standards Board
BAF	Board Assurance Framework
BSO	Business Services Organisation (Northern Ireland)
CCG	Clinical Commissioning Group
CHMS	Central Health and Miscellaneous Services
CHP	Community Health Partnerships
CIC	Community Interest Company
CNORIS	Clinical Negligence and Other Risks Indemnity Scheme (Scotland)
CNST	Clinical Negligence Scheme for Trusts
COS	Contracted Out Services (VAT)
CQC	Care Quality Commission
CQUIN	Commissioning for Quality and Innovation
CRL	Capital Resource Limit
CSR	Comprehensive Spending Review
CSU	Commissioning Support Unit
DEL	Departmental Expenditure Limit
DES	Directed Enhanced Services
DFT	Distance from Target
DHSSPS	Department of Health, Social Services and Public Safety (Northern Ireland)
DV	District Valuer
EFL	External Financing Limit
ENDPB	Executive Non-Departmental Body
EPS	Electronic Prescription Service
FCE	Finished Consultant Episode
FHS	Family Health Services
FMA	Financial Monitoring and Accounts form
FReM	Financial Reporting Manual
FRR	Financial Risk Rating
FT	NHS Foundation Trust
FTFF	Foundation Trust Financing Facility

GDP	Gross Domestic Product
GDS	General Dental Services (contract)
GMS	General Medical Services (contract)
GOS	General Ophthalmic Services
GP	General Practitioner
HCHS	Hospital and Community Health Services
HEAT	Health improvement, Efficiency and resources, Access, Treatment (targets – Scotland)
HEE	Health Education England
HEIG	Health Estates Investment Group (Northern Ireland)
HFMA	Healthcare Financial Management Association
HIW	Healthcare Inspectorate Wales
HRG	Healthcare Resource Group
HSC	Health and Social Care (Northern Ireland)
HSCB	Health and Social Care Board (Northern Ireland)
HWB	Health and Wellbeing Board
IASB	International Accounting Standards Board
IBP	Integrated Business Plan
ICT	Information Communications and Technology
IFRS	International Financial Reporting Standards
IPAG	Investment Policy and Appraisal Group (Wales)
ISD	Information and Statistics Division (Scotland)
ISTC	Independent Sector Treatment Centre
JHWS	Joint Health and Wellbeing Strategy
JSNA	Joint Strategic Needs Assessment
LCG	Local Commissioning Group (Northern Ireland)
LDP	Local Delivery Plan (Scotland)
LES	Local Enhanced Services
LETB	Local Education and Training Board
LHB	Local Health Board
LIFT	Local Improvement Finance Trust
LINKs	Local Involvement Networks
LPN	Local Professional Network
LSP	Local Strategic Partnership
MAQS	Materiality and Quality Score
MFF	Market Forces Factor
MPET	Multi Professional Education and Training
MRET	Marginal Rate Emergency Tariff
MUR	Medicine Use Review
NAO	National Audit Office
NED	Non-Executive Director
nGDS	'new' General Dental Services Contract
NHSLA	NHS Litigation Authority
NHS TDA	NHS Trust Development Authority
NIA	Northern Ireland Assembly
NIAO	Northern Ireland Audit Office
NICE	National Institute for Health and Care Excellence

NMS	New Medicine Service
NRAC	NHSScotland Resource Allocation Committee
NRCI	National Reference Cost Index
NSRC	National Schedule of Reference Costs
OECD	Organisation for Economic Co-operation and Development
OFR	Operating and Financial review
PAC	Public Accounts Committee
PASC	Public Administration Select Committee
PBC	Practice Based Commissioning
PBL	Prudential Borrowing Limit
PbR	Payment by Results
PCC	Patient and Client Council (Northern Ireland)
PCT	Primary Care Trust
PDC	Public Dividend Capital
PDS	Personal Dental Services (contract)
PES	Public Expenditure Survey
PFI	Private Finance Initiative
PFP	Prime Financial Policies
PHA	Public Health Agency (Northern Ireland)
PHE	Public Health England
PLICS	Patient Level Information and Costing Systems
PMS	Primary Medical Services
PSA	Public Service Agreement
QIPP	Quality, Innovation, Productivity and Prevention
QOF	Quality and Outcomes Framework
RAG	Red, Amber, Green (used for ratings)
RCI	Reference Cost Index
RPA	Review of Public Administration (Northern Ireland)
RQIA	Regulation and Quality Improvement Authority (Northern Ireland)
RRL	Revenue Resource Limit
SEO	Social Enterprise Organisation
SFE	Statement of Financial Entitlements
SFIs	Standing Financial Instructions
SGHSCD	Scottish Government Health and Social Care Directorate
SHA	Strategic Health Authority
SI	Statutory Instrument
SIFT	Service Increment for Teaching
SLA	Service Level Agreement
SLM	Service Line Management
SLR	Service Line Reporting
SO	Standing Orders
SOCI	Statement of comprehensive income
SOFA	Statement of Financial Activities
SORP	Statement of Recommended Practice
SUS	Secondary Uses Service
TAGRA	Technical Advisory Group on Resource Allocation (Scotland)
TCS	Transforming Community Services

TFA	Tripartite Formal Agreement
TME	Total Managed Expenditure
UDA	Unit of Dental Activity
WCC	World Class Commissioning
WGA	Whole of Government Accounts
WHSSC	Welsh Health Specialised Services Committee

Appendix 3: Glossary

Accountable/ Accounting Officer	Every NHS organisation has an 'Accountable' (or 'Accounting') Officer. This is a formal role conferred upon the organisation's 'Chief Officer' (usually the Chief Executive). In a CCG, the Chief Officer is either the 'lead manager' or the 'lead clinician.' The two terms are used because an Accounting Officer (for example in an FT or Department of Health) is directly accountable to Parliament whereas an Accountable Officer (for example, in a CCG or NHS trust) is responsible to an Accounting Officer of a government department who is in turn accountable to Parliament.
Accruals	An accounting concept that is designed to ensure that the accounts show all income and expenditure relating to the financial year regardless of whether cash has actually been received or paid. This means that in addition to payments and receipts of cash (and similar), adjustment is made for outstanding payments, debts to be collected, and stock (items bought, paid for but not yet used).
Amortisation	The process of charging the cost of an intangible asset such as a patent or software licence over its useful life as opposed to recording its cost as a single entry in the income and expenditure records. It is equivalent to depreciation for a tangible asset and (like depreciation) is an accounting charge so does not involve any cash outlay.
Assets	An item that has a value in the future. For example, a debtor (someone who owes money) is an asset, as they will in future pay. A building is an asset, because it houses activity that will provide a future income stream.
Audit	The process of validating the accuracy, completeness and adequacy of disclosure of financial records.
Benchmarking	The process of comparing objective information from similar activities or organisations to help identify the best way of providing a service or carrying out an activity. It can involve making comparisons within an organisation or with other organisations.
Block payment	A payment option used in contracts when PbR does not apply that involves commissioners paying healthcare providers a fixed amount of

money for access to a defined range and volume of service for the year ahead. The provider receives an amount of funding irrespective of the number of patients treated or the type of treatment provided.

Break-even

Income equals expenditure. It is important as an organisation cannot spend more than it has coming in and still be viable financially.

Business case

A formal process (in written form) for identifying the financial and qualitative implications of options for changing services and/or investing in capital.

Business plan

Also known as a service or operational plan, the business plan is the written end product of a process to identify the aims, objectives and resource requirements of an organisation over the next three to five year period. Generally business plans cover the forthcoming year in greater detail than those periods further in the future.

Capital

In most businesses, capital refers either to shareholder investment funds, or buildings, land and equipment owned by a business that has the potential to earn income in the future. The NHS uses this second definition, but adds a further condition – that the cost of the building/equipment must exceed a minimum threshold, normally £5,000. Capital is thus an asset (or group of functionally interdependent assets), with a useful life expectancy of greater than one year, whose cost exceeds £5,000.

Capital resource limit (CRL)

The CRL is an expenditure limit set each year for non-foundation organisations that limits the amount that can be spent on capital purchases. If net capital expenditure is less than the limit the target has been achieved.

Cost and volume payment

A payment option used in contracts when PbR does not apply that involves a fixed sum being paid for access to a defined range and volume of services. If there is a variation from the intended level of activity, there is a variation in payment levels according to a 'variation', or 'threshold agreement clause'.

Cost centre

Rather than record every cost incurred separately (which is not possible due to the sheer volume), costs are categorised into a number of distinct headings referred to as 'cost centres'. Usually cost centres are in line with an organisation's budget headings.

Cost improvement plan/programme (CIPs)

CIPs set out the savings that an organisation plans to make to reduce expenditure/increase efficiency. They are used to close the gap between the level of revenue received and expenditure incurred in any one year.

Cost per case payment A payment option used in contracts when PbR does not apply. For each episode or unit of care a payment to the service provider is agreed. This approach suits procedures that are infrequent, unpredictable, or can have significant cost variations.

Current assets Debtors, stocks, cash or similar – i.e. assets that are, or can be converted into, cash within the next twelve months.

Depreciation The process of charging the cost of an asset over its useful life as opposed to recording it as a single amount in the income and expenditure records when acquired. It is an 'accounting charge' (i.e. it does not involve any cash outlay) that recognises that the value of a capital asset is used up or 'consumed' over its useful life.

Direct costs Direct costs are costs that relate directly to a particular patient, activity or output and are 'driven' by it. For example, the cost of a radiographer is a direct cost to the radiology department, but an indirect cost to general surgery (as radiology serves several departments).

External financing limit (EFL) The EFL is an absolute financial duty. Its purpose is to control the cash expenditure of the NHS as a whole to the level agreed by Parliament in the public expenditure control totals. The EFL sets a limit on the level of cash that a non-foundation NHS trust may:

- draw from either external sources or its own cash reserves (a positive EFL) **OR**
- repay to external sources for capital borrowing (a negative EFL).

Fixed cost A cost that does not change as activity changes over a 12-month period – for example, depreciation.

General medical services Medical services provided by general practitioners (as opposed to other primary care providers such as dentists and community pharmacists).

Governance Governance (or corporate governance) is the system by which organisations are directed and controlled. It is concerned with how an organisation is run – how it structures itself and how it is led. Governance should underpin all that an organisation does. In the NHS this means it must encompass clinical, financial and organisational aspects.

Government Banking Service The Government Banking Service was established in April 2008 and is the banking shared service provider to government and the wider public sector. It is part of HM Revenue & Customs (HMRC) and incorporates the Office of HM Paymaster General (OPG) who had provided banking services to the public sector since 1836. It is responsible for holding the working balances of Government Departments and other public bodies in high-level accounts at the Bank of England.

Gross domestic product (GDP)	A measure of the value of national economic activity, GDP is the total money value of all final goods and services produced in an economy during a year.
Healthcare resource group (HRG)	The HRG is the 'currency' used to collate the costs of procedures/ diagnoses into common groupings to which tariffs can be applied.
Indirect costs	Costs that cannot be directly attributed to a particular patient, ward or cost centre but can be indirectly related to them. Such costs are usually collected at an aggregate level and are then allocated to individual cost centres.
Intangible asset	A capital asset that does not exist as a physical entity – for example, goodwill, brand value or some other right.
Overheads	The costs of support services that contribute to the effective running of the organisation but cannot be traced or easily related to a patient, activity or service and need to be allocated via an appropriate cost driver. For example, the total heating costs of a hospital may be apportioned to individual departments using floor area or cubic capacity.
Payment by results	The system for reimbursing healthcare providers in England for the costs of providing treatment. PbR is based around the use of a national tariff that links a pre-set price to a defined measure of output or activity.
Public dividend capital	A form of long-term government finance on which NHS organisations pay dividends to the Exchequer.
Reference costs	Reference costs record activity levels, unit cost data and average length of stay for a range of specified activities and are collected each year from all providers of health services (acute, community and paramedic) to NHS patients using NHS resources. The results are published each year in the National Schedule of Reference Costs.
Semi-fixed cost	Costs that are fixed for a given level of activity but change in steps when activity levels exceed or fall below these given levels. In other words, semi-fixed costs do not move with activity changes on a small scale, but 'jump' or 'step up' when a certain threshold is reached – for example, nursing staff.

Spending review A cyclical review undertaken by the Treasury to distribute public funding between the main governmental departments.

Statement of comprehensive income or statement of net expenditure One of the four primary statements in the accounts of NHS organisations, it shows the day to day revenue and expenditure for the organisation.

Statement of changes in taxpayers' equity One of the four primary statements in the accounts of NHS organisations. It shows how reserves have changed over the course of the year as a result of the organisation's financial performance.

Statement of financial position One of the four primary statements in the accounts of NHS organisations, it shows the assets, liabilities and equity as at a point in time, normally a month or year end.

Tangible asset A capital asset that physically exists such as land, buildings, equipment, fixtures and fittings.

Variable cost A cost that varies proportionately with changes in activity – for example, drugs and consumables costs.

Variance The difference between budgeted and actual income and/or expenditure. Variances are an accounting tool used to analyse the cause of over/under spends with a view to proposing rectifying action.

Working capital Working capital is the money and assets that an organisation can call upon to finance its day-to-day operations (it is the difference between current assets and liabilities and is reported in the statement of financial position as net current assets (liabilities)). If working capital dips too low, organisations risk running out of cash and may need a working capital loan to smooth out the troughs.

Whole of Government Accounts The consolidated set of financial statements for the UK public sector. It brings together the audited accounts of over 1,500 organisations across the public sector, including central government departments, local authorities, devolved administrations, the health service, academies and public corporations, in order to produce a comprehensive, accounts-based picture of the fiscal position in any one year.